PALEO FOR BEGINNERS

*Start Your Ideal 7 Day Paleo Diet Plan
for Beginners to Lose Weight in 21 Days!*

OLIVIA ROSE

TABLE OF CONTENTS

INTRODUCTION

Dear reader,

I firstly want to express my thanks to you for buying and downloading the book *"Paleo Diet For Beginners: Start Your Ideal Paleo Diet For Beginners & Lose Weight In 21 Day!- Over 50 Recipes Included"*.

I also want to tell you that you're awesome for wanting to lose weight with a Paleo Diet. This book contains proven steps and strategies on how to lose those stubborn excess pounds and live a healthier life with the help of the Paleo diet.

The prehistoric men lived longer, healthier, and more active lives during their time. It was attributed to the diet, lifestyle, and simple living that they practiced. With all the advanced technologies the modern man is enjoying today, one would have thought that going back to the Paleolithic era is not the answer to weight and health problems. It is.

Here are some benefits of the Paleo Diet

Rich in nutrients
One misconception about Paleo diet is that it only emphasizes on fat and protein. However, by eliminating processed food, you can add more vegetables, fruit, seeds and healthy fat in your diet. Paleo diet encourages the consumption of foods rich in nutrients and minerals. Eliminating grain in your diet can also improve your digestion and nutrient absorption.

Weight loss
Many people experience weight loss and muscle growth while on the Paleo diet. This is the reason why many athletes choose the Paleo diet. The diet can also improve your metabolic process and promote better sleep.

Reduce bloat
Paleo diet is rich in fiber. If you pair this with adequate water consumption and reduced salt intake, it can help reduce bloating. Also, the diet can help keep the gut healthy.

No more hangry
'Hangry' is a term that combines hungry and angry. It is also a symptom of hyperglycemia which happens when your blood sugar drops too low. Its symptoms include fatigue, irritability and foggy brain. The Paleo diet is rich in nutrient dense food that can keep blood sugar stable.

Rich in healthy fats
The Paleo diet makes use of a lot of healthy fat sources including seafood, meat, coconut and butter. These fats are essential in keeping your heart, brain and skin healthy.

Going back to the basics of consuming natural and fresh foods, such as the ancestors did, has proven to be one of the answers to everyone's search for weight loss and a higher quality of life. There is more to the Paleo diet than food, though.

Find out the solution and enjoy a healthier and leaner you, all in 21 days!

Thanks again for downloading this book, I hope you enjoy it!

CHAPTER ONE:
PALEO DIET: AN INTRODUCTION

Weight problems have been in existence since time immemorial. The main culprit of this problem is diet. Other contributing factors include lack of exercise, genetics, certain medications, lack of rest and sleep, and pre-existing medical conditions (such as Cushing's syndrome, hypothyroidism, and Prader-Willi syndrome).

Man has over and over again tried to combat weight problems. People keep on finding new ways and means to win the battle against weight disorders. With all the technologies available at man's disposal, the answer to the problem was found by going back hundreds of thousands of years ago, specifically during the Paleolithic era.

Brief History of Paleo Diet

More than 100 years ago, a man by the name of Joseph Knowles decided to try and live like our ancestors for two months. He stayed in the wilderness and imitated the diet of the so-called "hunter-gatherer people" during the Paleolithic era, the time before the development of agriculture. Although Knowles did not coin the term Paleo diet, he initiated the theory of alternative diet and healthier life by following the dietary regimen of our prehistoric ancestors.

Dr. Walter Voegtin gave the term "Paleo diet" during the 1970s. He was a gastroenterologist and an author. He believed that the Paleo diet would provide today's mankind the highest level of health as it did with our ancestors. The longer lifespan, strength and absence of modern day diseases of the people during this era were attributed to the diet that they observed during their time. Practicing the same dietary regimen would benefit the people of today, very much the same way it did before.

However, the idea of the Paleo diet was not met with enthusiasm during the 70's. After much studies and analyses by other health experts though, this diet slowly gained popularity through the years. Today, people are very much aware of the wonders of this diet when it comes to losing weight and achieving general health and wellbeing. It even became Google's most searched method for weight loss in 2013.

What Is the Paleo Diet?

The Paleo diet is known by other names such as the cavemen diet, hunter-gatherer diet, and Stone Age diet. The concept behind this diet came from the premise that what worked for the forefathers' health would also work for today's population. Adoption of the eating habits, food selections, and lifestyle of our prehistoric ancestors are the main objectives.

Since the Paleolithic era came before the age of agriculture, there was no cultivation of crops yet. The Paleolithic ancestors gathered foods only. They did not raise animals, too. They just fished and hunted animals for meat. The Paleo diet of today therefore consists of foods that could have been hunted and gathered only by prehistoric man.

Included in the diet are mostly fish and meat and products of plants such as vegetables, fruits and nuts. As there were no ways to process foods back then, all processed foods are to be avoided in this diet. The only sugar that is allowed is honey. Salt, on the other hand, is limited. Off-limits are the grains, dairy products and all canned, cured, smoked, and preserved products.

The Completeness of the Paleo Diet

A big factor for the gaining popularity of this diet is its completeness when it comes to planning a menu. The ingredients are varied and they are readily available at the local groceries. The recipes are plenteous and are very easy to prepare and make. The dishes are delicious. You would not feel as though you are sacrificing in the name of health, as some health diets do. The followers of the Paleo diet would not have the cravings and feelings of deprivation that usually accompany those who are following other diets designed to make one healthier and leaner.

Another big factor is its success rate for those who are trying to lose weight. The following reasons are given why the Paleo diet is highly recommended for weight watchers.

1. The compliance to the diet is high. The Paleo dieters usually abide to the dietary restrictions set to them. This "phenomenon" could be attributed to the delicious recipes and the variety of food selections that the Paleo diet offers. Not to mention, total absence of processed foods in the diet is tantamount to hundreds of calories deductions.

2. The Paleo diet is not just about what you take in. It is also about what you do not take in at certain periods of time. Fasting in between meals are sometimes done to simulate the imagined "lean times" that the prehistoric people have encountered while hunting for their foods. Fasting allows the gastrointestinal system to rest and it helps in reducing the amount of food needed to make you feel full. As you habitually do this, there is an increased tendency to get used to eating small amount of food at each meal, leading to the desired weight loss.

3. Aside from the effects of their food intake, Paleo diet followers also experience success in losing those excess weights as they usually engage in strenuous activities or exercises as they diet. This is equivalent to the efforts of the Paleolithic ancestors as they hunted down animals. Weight lifting exercise is the parallel activity for carrying the heavy animals after they were killed. The exercises cause the weight loss

and the toned muscles, making Paleo dieters feel and look good.

The Paleo diet is a success because of the following reasons: it is simple, doable, and effective. Weight loss is achievable within three weeks and great health is possible for good with continuous implementation of this diet in your lifestyle.

The Evolution of Paleo Diet

Originally, the Paleo diet followed a strict list of what is allowed and what is not. Throughout the years, however, the Paleo diet has evolved. Several versions of the Paleo diet now include some modern foods, drinks and ingredients that science has found to be healthy. For instance, wine can be taken in small amount even when you are in Paleo diet. Studies have shown that quality red wine is good for health because it is high in antioxidants and other beneficial nutrients. You would also see some Paleo recipes with dark chocolates in them. It has been established how healthy and nutritious dark chocolates are.

Previously, strict Paleo diets of before would not allow the use of utensils and appliances that the prehistoric people did not use. That too has evolved and has been modified. Today, there are baked Paleo desserts today when you know for a fact that electricity was not yet discovered during that time, how much more the ovens. There are also smoothies, shakes and drinks that are included in the Paleo diet nowadays albeit there were no food processors or blenders before.

The Future of Paleo Diet

Although the Paleo diet is only a century old, the future of this dietary regimen is bright and definite. Studies and researches are continuous as more and more people are utilizing this diet. Even with the rapid advancement of technology, the so-called "evolutionary theory" of the Paleo diet trend has remained strong and stable. One can conclusively state that the Paleo diet is here to stay.

CHAPTER TWO:
PALEO DIET AND ITS HOLISTIC BENEFITS TO THE MODERN MAN

When one is uncertain if a particular food is allowed in the Paleo diet, one just has to determine whether that food is processed or not. All processed foods are not permitted in this regimen. The Paleo diet encourages fresh vegetable and fruits instead. With this restriction alone, you have saved yourself from diseases, obesity and bad effects that these processed foods can give you.

The Dangers Of Processed Foods

It has been medically and scientifically proven what these so-called "slow killers" can do to your body. Here are some information about processed foods that might help you appreciate the Paleo diet more:

➤ Processed foods are known to disrupt the blood sugar level due to its high sugar content and high content of refined carbohydrates. This makes a person prone to endocrine diseases, with Diabetes Mellitus as the most common.

➤ Processed foods can make you overweight or worse, obese as you tend to eat more because satiety or feeling of fullness is not felt early. It has this false feel-good effect every time you eat, causing you to eat more.

➤ Processed foods make one susceptible to diseases such as cancer, allergic reactions and kidney problems due to its artificial ingredients. Food preservatives or additives such as Butylated hydroxyanisole (BHA), have been found to have a strong link to these diseases.

➤ Addictive property is discovered among processed

foods. This makes it difficult for one to easily give up chips, sodas and other junk foods.

➢ Processed foods have low nutritional value. The body's needs for nutrients, vitamins and minerals are not being supplied.

➢ These are also typically low in fiber. Problems in excretory system (the one responsible for the removal of waste products of the body) usually exist because of limited fiber in the diet.

➢ On the other hand, processed foods are high in trans fats. This is one factor for having cardiovascular diseases in the form of atherosclerosis or in layman's term, formation of blockages in the arterial walls as caused by accumulation of plaques, due to intake of foods with trans fat.

Man is a bio-psychosocial being. Whereas most diets are focused on the physical aspect only, the Paleo diet covers the totality of man, thereby providing holistic benefits. Here are some of the beneficial effects of this prehistoric diet to the modern man of today.

Effects of Paleo Diet in the Physical Aspect

1. *It makes you healthier and less prone to disease.* Physically speaking, the benefits of the Paleo diet has been established already by simply removing processed foods in the picture. The Paleo diet favors consumption of fresh vegetables and fruits. Most people are already aware of the benefits of eating fresh vegetables and fruits. To name just a few, prevention of hypertension, heart diseases, gastrointestinal disorders, and even cancer have been linked to increased consumption of vegetables and fruits.

2. *Paleo diet has been effective in making many people shed off excess pounds.* Not only because unprocessed

foods burn more calories to eat and digest but also because this diet is not just focused on food intake but also on exercise and fasting between meals, as previously discussed. The combination of food allowed in this diet has a direct effect on how the body processes the food. This will be discussed fully in later chapters.

3. *One is more energized and active.* Physically, you tend to be stronger and more active with Paleo diet. The proteins and fats included in the diet allow one to increase in physical undertakings minus the feelings of tiredness and easy fatigability.

4. *Paleo dieters look and feel better.* The weight loss, toned muscles, overall light feeling contribute to enhanced physical outcomes. One looks younger too because of the anti-aging properties of some foods included in the Paleo diet.

These are just some of the benefits of this dietary regimen to one's physical attributes. There are more benefits identified and this time, in other aspects of man. This is where Paleo diet tops other health diet regimens. Unlike other diet fads, Paleo diet encompasses man's whole being.

Psychological Benefits of Paleo Diet

The psychology of man includes the mental, cognitive and emotional states. Paleo diet encourages people to utilize all natural resources and processes rather than depend on technology and artificial and processed stuff. With all things being equal, eating healthy foods make one healthy. And when one is healthy, the mental, cognitive and emotional components are also affected positively. Paleo diet has caused the following enhancements on the psychological aspect of man.

1. What you eat affects what you feel. Let's focus on the emotional aspect first. Processed and other unhealthy

foods give you the temporary "high" and "false good-feel" effects for several minutes to an hour. Afterwards, the long-term effects of low nutrition and inadequate supply of essential minerals and vitamins could lead to depression and anxiety. Studies have shown that people who consume more sodas and chips have a higher tendency to be depressed. Meanwhile, healthy foods can cause real and lasting feel-good effects and overall happiness and positivity.

2. Foods affect your mind and mental health. Healthy foods cause the brain's tissues to be protected from damage and attacks of harmful bacteria. At the same time, healthy foods provide the needed nutrients by the brain for it to thrive and survive. When one feeds on foods that are good for the brain, increased mental alertness, better memories and improved comprehension are achieved.

3. Absence of medical conditions brought about by inappropriate food intake could increase positive outlook and response to life in general.

There is a connection between what you eat and how you feel, understand and think. The Paleo diet does not claim to make one stress-free but it helps in increasing one's ability to respond to life's stresses on a more positive note.

Benefits of the Paleo Diet on the Social Aspect of Man

Standing on the premises of evolutionary theory, the Paleo diet promotes simplicity and self-dependency. Going back to the basics, leaving the thrills and frills of modernity, is one beauty of the Paleo diet. The Paleo dieters capture this ideal and aids in making them more sociable and likeable.

1. What you eat also affects how you relate to others. When one feels good about oneself, that sensation is transferred to other people. There is a heightened tendency to be nicer and friendlier to others.

2. Your overall physical health affects your activities and social life too. Physical strength brought about by healthy foods makes a person more inclined towards productivity and efficiency. Relationships also improve when people do not have any physical discomforts that could make them more irritable and impatient.
3. Some followers of the Paleo dieters simulated the simple living of the prehistoric people, cutting down on materialism and worldliness. Social wise, they have adapted the simple ways and manners of the Paleo ancestors and have won more acquaintances in the process.

There is indeed a connection between your food consumption and overall personality. A better you is just a by-product of a healthier you. The saying "you are what you eat" summarizes this point of discussion.

It is now time to discover the many recipes and meal plans that the Paleo diet offers. Read on!

CHAPTER THREE:
THE 21-DAY CHALLENGE

Why 21 days?

Previous researches reveal that a minimum timeframe of 3 weeks or 21 days is needed for a new habit to become a lifestyle. The same number of days is applicable for incorporating a new diet into a person's daily routine. To replace the old mindset, a person needs to establish something new by practicing it every day for at least three consecutive weeks. If you pass the 21-day mark, that is a promising note that you are on your way to making it permanently a part of your life.

Requirements To Participate In This Challenge

Anybody can decide to engage in this dietary program with the intention to lose weight in 21 days. However, with no real dedication and commitment, a person can end up unsuccessful and miss the opportunity to experience a better health and an upgraded quality of life. This program guarantees 100% success only to those who are truly and wholeheartedly devoted to continuing the dietary regimen.

Before you proceed and start the program, read the following requirements and decide for yourself if the Paleo diet is for you.

1) You understand what the Paleo diet is all about. One can give his or her whole heart to something that one fully knew well. If you've just heard about the Paleo diet from friends and family members but did not study this yourself, your motivation to complete it would not be that strong. One has to involve the body, mind, will, and emotion to ensure success.

2) Inform your primary health care provider. The decision to change your diet and lifestyle would need the approval of your doctor especially if you are currently undergoing therapies or medications because of an existing medical condition. Visit and inform your doctor of your intention to follow the Paleo diet. A thorough physical examination and check up may be required prior to observance of this diet.

   a) As with all other changes in diet, the body tends to react and present withdrawal symptoms especially in the first week of the regimen. For instance, there may be intense cravings for foods that are not allowed in the diet (soda and chips top the list). There may be some behavioral changes at first like irritability or impatience. At first, you may seem like grumpy. Sometimes, shaking of fingers is observed. All these are the body's natural responses to change. Allow some margin for these reactions.

   b) If the physical reactions are seemingly out of the norm, do not hesitate to call your doctor. You may also stop the diet while you wait for the go-signal of your physician.

3) Believe in yourself. The biggest factor for the success of the Paleo diet is YOU. Your full cooperation is required to accomplish the initial 21-day challenge. Believe that you can and you will finish and be successful in this endeavor. Have faith in yourself, in your ability, and in your willpower. Have a positive mental attitude towards the dietary program. Always remind yourself that you have what it takes to be a success in this.

4) Write down you vision and target. How much weight do you want to shed off? When do you plan to accomplish this? What are the things that you need to do before you can fulfill all the necessary things for the program? Have several copies of the vision and target in places where you can see them such as in the bathroom mirror, your wallet, cellphone, tabletop or diary. It is a must that you can visualize yourself achieving the target. As early as

now, picture yourself completing the program and enjoying a healthier, leaner, and lighter body.

5) Inform you family and significant others of your intention to shift to Paleo diet. Why is there a need to do this? For the following reasons:

   a) The one in charge of the food preparation in your home should be instructed on what meal to cook for you. There should be coordination among the family members.

   b) If you are living alone, it will still be beneficial to involve your family, friends or even co-workers to this. There may be times that you would be in a gathering and they would understand why you are not eating certain foods. Or, awkwardness could be eliminated when they give or surprise you with food and you cannot eat it. They would know what to prepare for you.

   c) Family members are great cheerleaders. There would be times that you might feel that you just want to give up and just return to your previous diet and life. Your family can boost your determination by encouraging you to continue. Studies show that those who have strong support system are more bound to succeed than those who do not have.

6) Initially, keep a list of what is allowed or not for you. It is better to be sure than to repeat the process over again because of an error. This tip could also save you time when you do your grocery shopping.

7) Basically, Paleo diet is about food consumption but that is not all to it. Incorporate into your lifestyle those habits of the Paleo man like exertion of efforts similar to that of hunting (in the form of exercise), intermittent fasting (during lean time and winter season of the prehistoric man), early to bed & early to rise schedule (as there was no electricity and any form of entertainment yet and easy simple living (less stressful life). These are great helps to achieve your desired weight and healthier body.

Commitment to the 21-day Challenge

There is a guarantee of weight loss and a better health. However, there is also a certainty of having moments when you feel like you would not be able to finish and comply with the dietary modification and just give up.

There are many factors that can make you a success in this undertaking. However, the main factor is you. Your total participation and cooperation would divide the line between success and defeat. This dietary program has been tried and tested by millions of people. On the other hand, it has been tried and has caused disappointments to others too. The bottom line is this: technically, it is not about the diet. It is all about you.

Therefore, commit today that you would commit your heart, mind, and body to adhering to the Paleo diet. Look within yourself. Be reminded that everything you need to overcome the challenge of being overweight is already deposited in the inside of you. All you have to do is to unleash the potential already within. Do not just mentally assent to this truth but embrace it with everything you got.

If you have a sincere intention of completing the program and even continuing it after the 3-week timeframe, then do not just verbalize it, do not just think about it, do not just dream about it. Make it official by signing the Commitment Form below. Look for a family member or a significant other to be your witness. You could have more witnesses if you prefer. They would serve as your partners in your objective to complete the regimen. You would be accountable to them in this project by always updating them of your progress, asking for their assistance during attacks of "giving-up" moments and celebrating with them in your hour of victory. Sign this form today and you are halfway to success already. Sign now!

Commitment Form

I, (complete name) _____, hereby commit this day (date)_____to abide by the instructions and mechanisms of the Paleo diet, with my whole heart, body and mind. I commit to give my best and exert all efforts to ensure complete compliance to the dietary modifications that I would do. I pledge to fulfill all the basic requirements stated above to warrant the success of this regimen. Paleo diet is not just another health diet fad for me.

I would complete the 21-day plan for me. I am set to continue the diet even after the three-week time is over to guarantee maintenance of the expected change.

Sign here :
Witness' Signature :
Date:

Congratulations! You are indeed halfway to your destination. A quick reminder of the requirements: study and learn about the Paleo diet, inform your primary health care provider and family or friends, believe in yourself, write down the vision and target, keep a list, and perform other healthy habits as well.

CHAPTER FOUR:
THE BASICS OF THE PALEO DIET

The Paleo diet is designed after the diet of the prehistoric man during the Paleolithic era. That was the time before the development of agriculture. So the Paleo man did not plant and cultivate crops. They just gathered from their surroundings the available plant products for consumption. The Paleo ancestors did not raise animals either. They hunted whatever animals they could hunt during those days. They fished. That's why this diet is also called the "hunter-gatherer" diet.

The main thing about this dietary regimen is this principle: there are no processed foods allowed. Consume whole, unprocessed foods that may have been available during the Paleolithic era.

What are the foods allowed and restricted in Paleo diet?

What is beautiful about the Paleo diet is the long list of allowed foods for consumption. Paleo dieters do not have to undergo severe "sacrifices" by giving up on their beloved foods. The shift in the diet would not really be that overwhelming. Plus, the ingredients are all readily available in all grocery stores unlike some health diets where most of the ingredients are out of this world.

Here is a summary of "what's to eat" under the Paleo diet.

Allowed foods

> ➢ Almost all fresh vegetables
> ➢ Fresh fruits
> ➢ Grass-produced meats

➢ Fish/other sea foods
➢ Seeds
➢ Nuts
➢ Eggs
➢ Herbs and spices
➢ Oils and fats that are considered healthy
➢ Dark chocolates (dairy-free)
➢ Quality red wine

Here is a comprehensive list of the allowed foods as your guideline in your 21-day diet.

Fresh Vegetables
Almost all things that our Paleolithic ancestors harvested are considered as goodies such as the following:

- spinach
- asparagus
- artichoke hearts
- broccoli
- zucchini
- celery
- cabbage
- okra
- eggplants
- avocado
- parsley
- green onions
- Brussels sprouts

Although butternut squash, yam, potatoes, sweet potatoes, beets, and acorn squash are under the category of fresh veggies, consumption of these vegetables are encouraged to be limited to once or twice a week only. These are considered starchy vegetables.However, if you are training and exercising vigorously, then the starchy veggies are great for energy replacements.

Fresh vegetables can be eaten raw, grilled or steamed. Refrain from frying them as much as possible.

Fresh fruits

Just like with the fresh vegetables, imagine the prehistoric ancestors picking fruits and eating them right away. Fruits are high in fructose content (a form of sugar) so try to limit fruit intake. However, if you really like them,you can eat up to 3 servings per day.Fruits are still better choice than chips for snacks. Choose organic fruits. Avoid canned, dried and preserved fruits. Here are some examples:

- All berries
- Apples
- Peaches
- Papaya
- Plums
- Lychees
- Mango
- Lemons
- Watermelons
- Avocado
- Grapes
- Tangerines
- Lime
- Cantaloupe
- Figs
- Oranges
- Pineapple
- Guavas
- Kiwi

Bananas are starchy too so do not eat so much of them unless you are exercising hard. Fruits are great for snacks and salad additions. Eat them fresh as much as possible.

Grass-produced meats

Almost all meats are included in the Paleo diet. Thus, it is believed our hunter-gatherer ancestors did not suffer from atherosclerosis or coronary artery heart diseases brought about by meat consumption. Basically all meats are good to eat except of course if they are processed. And just like with all diets, moderation in consumption is recommended.

- chicken
- turkey
- pork
- steak
- veal
- grass-fed beef
- lamb
- venison steaks
- ox or bison
- rabbit
- goat
- deer
- kangaroos
- emu
- wild boar
- elk
- goose
- ostrich
- snakes
- reindeer
- quail
- turtles
- bears

Great list, isn't it? You will never run out of menus and dishes with a list this long.

Fish and other Seafood

If you could find them in the water, if they could swim, and if they have fins, you can eat them. They are considered as Paleo.

- Red snapper
- Bass
- Salmon
- Sardines
- Shark
- Sunfish
- Halibut
- Mackerel
- Tuna
- Tilapia
- Swordfish
- Walleye
- Lobsters
- Crabs
- Eels
- Shrimps
- Clams
- Oysters
- Milkfish
- Scallops
- Crayfish
- Crawfish

These are just some of the allowed fish and seafood and yet, these are mouth-watering already. These are great for sushi, soups, and main dishes. These are also good sources of omega 3, the essential fatty acids that the body needs.

Seeds and Nuts

Great for snacks and salads, these seeds and nuts are must have.

- hazelnuts
- pecans
- almonds
- pine nuts
- cashews
- sunflower seeds
- pumpkin seeds
- macadamia nuts
- walnuts

Take note, however, that peanuts are not considered as nuts and are therefore not included in the Paleo diet.

Eggs

Since some oils are not included in the healthy options, avoid frying eggs. There are also many incidences of medical conditions being acquired from eating raw eggs, so refrain from doing that.

- Chicken
- Duck
- Goose
- Quail

Herbs and Spices

Another beautiful thing about the Paleo diet is the inclusion of herbs and spices which make the dishes tastier and more delectable. Here are tips when buying your spices to ensure freshness: buy them whole and grind them yourself. You could avail of an affordable coffee grinder, which you could use specifically for spices. For larger spices such as cinnamon and nutmeg, use a microplane grater instead. Buy your spices in bulk. You would need these most of the time anyway, and it is cheaper that way. If there are Asian food stores in your area, buy your spices from them. Asians love to use herbs and spices in their dishes so you can expect fresher supplies of spices in their stores.

As expected, garlic and onions top the list. Here are other spices you can use.

- chili powder
- cinnamon
- cumin
- cardamom
- paprika
- nutmeg
- thyme
- rosemary
- all peppers

Paleo dieters love to have their own garden for their herbs. For those who do not possess green thumbs, you could always avail of these in grocery stores.

- cilantro or coriander
- celery
- bay leaf
- ginger
- clove
- basil
- turmeric
- parsley
- chives
- fennel
- oregano
- sage
- sesame

You would never want your dishes without these healthy herbs and spices again.

Healthy Oils and Fats
These ingredients can help you with your needed energy

when you are undergoing the Paleo diet and its recommended exercises. They are also great for salads to mix with your vegetables and fruits.

- Macadamia oil
- Olive oil
- Coconut oil
- Avocado oil
- Grass fed sources of butter

Other foods that are included

Honey is allowed. Sea salt and Himalayan salts can be used too. Clarified butter or Ghee is also used as a substitute for regular butters.

New additions

Aside from this list, addition to the modified Paleo diet's allowed foods now include dark chocolate. The recommended ones are the dairy free and 70% cocoa. You could bake them, make them as shakes or ice creams, or just eat them on their own.

For wine lovers, quality red wines are now part of the Paleo diet. The wine was found to be beneficial for health. The recommended amount though is a glass for a day only. That is just the enough amount that one can use for socializing.

Short Reminder

These are the allowed foods for Paleo diet. The list is quite long, if you would notice. Either you carry a list with you, because you cannot just totally depend on your memory with this, or you could stick to this principle: it's Paleo when the foods are unprocessed, unsweetened, and not fried.

CHAPTER FIVE:
GOODBYE TO THESE – RESTRICTED FOODS IN THE PALEO DIET

For most new followers of the Paleo diet, here is where the challenge starts – bidding goodbye to their old favorites. Some even go to the extent of consuming these in great amount and frequency before they start the diet. Others had withdrawal symptoms because their bodies were so used to these foods that adjustment without these took a little bit longer than the usual.

A quick look to "what's not to eat" under the Paleo diet.

Restricted foods

- All processed foods and drinks (candies, sodas, chips, junk foods)
- Grains
- Refined sugar and artificial sweeteners
- Dairy
- Legumes
- Refined vegetable oils
- Margarine and trans fat
- Salt

Check if your favorite foods are included in this comprehensive list of foods to avoid when in Paleo regimen.

All Processed Foods and Drinks

There is no going around this. Say goodbye to excess weights and poor nutrition by bidding your farewells to these. Previously you have learned the bad effects of processed foods in your health. Admittedly though, many struggle in this area because of the following reasons:

1. Processed foods taste so good. Do not be tricked. Salty foods such as chips, French fries, and pizzas tend to be eaten in quantity. Aside from the additives put on these that make them more palatable to the tongue, they also tend to fill the stomach at a later time. This means you eat a lot but you do not feel full so the tendency is to eat and eat some more. With little or nutritional value at all, these foods would just cause a person to increase in weight.

2. Since these foods are usually high in sugar too, the taste buds are delighted. Sweets have the highest taste recognition threshold. The brain perceives it as rewards. That's why one feels happier when one eats something sugary and sweet such as chocolates and ice cream. However, the sugar blood level is disrupted and proneness to metabolic and endocrine disorders are increasing in numbers because of this culprit – sugar.

3. Processed foods have addictive properties. Getting it out of the system would really require some effort and determination. The earlier you get out however, the better your adjustment without them. That is why, kids today should be trained to avoid sugary foods as early as possible.

4. Processed foods are everywhere! It is so much easier to shop for processed foods than look for healthy foods. With the preservatives that these foods contain, they also spoil quite later than real foods. They even look more attractive. So when it comes to convenience for the consumers, nothing can beat processed foods.

Even when one goes to fine restaurants or fast foods, there are limited dishes that one can find in the menu. There will, definitely, no Paleo dishes being offered.

Here they are. All foods that are chemically processed and

contain artificial flavorings and color, have refined sugars and preservatives would fit the description of processed foods. Therefore, the list could fill in the whole ebook. You would not be able to memorize them. To make it easier for you, use this as a guideline instead.

- Artificial ingredients – check the labels for tartrazine, aspartame, sucralose, and synthetic dyes and such. Or better yet, just ditch those with artificial colorings. Anyway, the reason they put coloring is to hide something about the food or just to make it more attractive. You do not need these.
- Canned goods – these are usually high in preservatives and salts.
- Foods from fast food chain stores –these taste good because they are usually loaded with additives.
- Those with low fat or fat-free labels. These can be deceiving as most consider them as healthy. Yes, they are healthy when you talk about the fats but in terms of sugar or additives, they tend to be high. This is done to make up for the bad taste of fat-free foods.
- Smoke, cured, preserved meats such as hotdogs, nuggets, chorizo, pepperoni, salami, jerky just to name a few.

Stick to the fresh and organic produces as much as possible.

Grains

Another challenge for the Paleo dieters is the removal of grains in the diet. Anything that has grain on it is considered as *un*Paleo and not to be taken.

- cereals
- pasta
- bread (muffins, sandwiches, toasts)
- crackers and biscuits
- oatmeal

- pancakes
- beers
- wheat

Take this thought to heart: the Paleo man survived without these, you could too. Here's good news however. The Paleo people have come up with their own versions of grains so you could still enjoy your pancakes, pastas and other grain-filled foods, Paleo style.

Refined sugar and artificial sweeteners

Much has been said about the hazards of sugar to the body. You could thank the Paleo diet later on when most of the people you know are suffering from medical conditions such as Diabetes, Candidiasis, and kidney problems because of sugar.

Sodas, chocolates, and sugars should be avoided at all cost. For artificial sweeteners, check the label for the following and do not purchase foods with these:

- Aspartame
- Glycerol
- Maltitol
- Lactitol
- Isomalt
- Solbitol
- Sucralose

Dairy

The Paleo ancestors consumed milk only in their infant stage, and the only milk they consumed were their mothers' milk. Afterwards, they were no more dairy products for them, but it did them so much good back then. It would do the modern man good too to refrain from consuming foods with dairy products included in the ingredients. Examples are:

- regular milk
- cheese
- butters
- creams

Legumes

Legumes are considered "un-Paleo." Here is a complete list of legumes not suitable to be eaten during the Paleo regimen.

- All beans (black, broad, fava, kidney beans, garbanzos, lima, navy, horse beans, pinto, adzuki, mung beans, red, green, white and string beans).
- Peas such as black eyed peas, snowpeas, chickpeas and sugar snap peas)
- Peanuts and other products with them such as peanut butter, peanut oil and candies with peanuts)
- Miso
- Lentils
- Soybeans and all its derivatives (tofu)

Refined vegetable oils

- corn oil
- rice bran oil
- wheat germ oil
- cottonseed oil
- foods such as mayonnaise which is rich in these oils.

Others

Margarine and trans fat, table salt and alcoholic beverages such as vodka, rum, beers, tequila and whiskey are not allowed too. Fruit juices, energy drinks and sodas are definitely "no-no" to this regimen as they contain high glucose, artificial flavors and additives and coloring. Plus, they are totally zero nutrients.

Last words on the restricted foods

Yes, admittedly, Paleo diet has a long list of "what's not to eat".However, the long-term positive effects of being without these foods far outweigh the delicious tastes of these unhealthy foods. Yes, there will be days when you'll crave and miss these restricted foods so much that you would want to give up on Paleo diet.Stop and take a deep breath. Imagine how lean, fit and healthy you would be if you would continue with the regimen. After several minutes, you will be surprised to find the cravings and longings to eat those foods gone.

Read on

It's time to find out the delicious meals that are available. In the next chapter, you will have a sample meal plan for a week plus easy to do recipes with nutritional information and photos. Have fun!

CHAPTER SIX:
SAMPLE PALEO MEALS FOR A WEEK

Planning is a vital key to your Paleo diet success. It would also make your grocery time a lot faster when you have a list of things to buy. Add more fruits and vegetables when you shop that you can use as substitute snacks when hunger pangs strike. Your stomach would need a little more time to adjust so once in a while, you would feel the urge to eat more. It's better to be ready than to overeat afterwards due to the feeling of deprivation.

So as not to overwhelm you, try not to do a drastic change in your diet. Make the shift gradual. Here is just a sample meal for a week. You have the liberty to follow this or to mix and match recipes and make your own meal plan. Remember, the first three weeks are crucial. Try to stick to the plan as much as possible. After the three weeks, the body is expected to have conformed to the change and would not react as much to the change.

Once you have decided on your 7-day meal plan, try to make several copies of the plan. Place one on your refrigerator. This is to stop you from taking foods you are not supposed to eat. It would actually be more helpful if you could remove all the restricted foods in the ref but if this is not possible (for instance, you are still living with your family), then a note on the ref's door would at least remind you of your new diet.

Place a copy of the plan on your person too. Just in case you would not be at home to prepare your meals, you could still follow the meal by ordering food or buying foods with similar ingredients and preparation.

7-day Meal Plan Sample

Monday
Breakfast: 2 eggs and bacon
Lunch: Grilled chicken strips and asparagus
Dinner: Salmon and avocado

Tuesday
Breakfast: Paleo Pancakes with strawberries or blueberries
Lunch: Salad with romaine lettuce and fruits
Dinner: Rotisserie chicken with vegetables on the side

Wednesday
Breakfast: Green smoothie (kiwi or kale)
Lunch: Strip steak and mixed vegetables
Dinner: Hamburger patty and spinach

Thursday
Breakfast: Fruits
Lunch: Grilled chicken with vegetable salad
Dinner: Grilled tuna with celery and herbs

Friday
Breakfast: Tomato and egg stir fry and apples
Lunch: Strip steak and mixed veggies
Dinner: Paleo spaghetti

Saturday
Breakfast: Leftover Paleo spaghetti
Lunch: citrus beef salad stir fry
Dinner: lemon and garlic scallops

Sunday
Breakfast: coconut milk smoothie and a bowl of berries
Lunch: citrus roast chicken with sweet potato fries
Dinner: beef goulash

Note: In between meals and when you feel hungry, you do not have to be a martyr and go on empty stomach. You can have snacks of nuts, fresh fruits, hard boiled eggs, pork rinds, smoothies, shakes, desserts, soups, dark chocolates and other Paleo snacks.

Take note, however, that fasting in between days and meals is also encouraged. Can you imagine the Paleo man having loads of foods in their caves? Maybe not. There were lean seasons during their time. So there was a possibility that they fasted on several occasions. Intermittent fasting has been studied to be a good way to lose weight too. Plus while on fast, it allows the different body systems to rest and recuperate.

If you are hard on the budget, there is good news for you. Paleo diet can be done even when the budget is tight. Here is a sample meal plan for those who would not be able to avail of steaks, scallops or expensive seafood for now.

A budgeted 7-day meal plan

Monday
Breakfast: omelets
Lunch: apple cider pork with rosemary
Dinner: strip chicken and mixed veggies

Tuesday
Breakfast: tomato quiche and fruits
Lunch: big romaine lettuce salad with tuna
Dinner: Smoky roasted butternut soup

Wednesday
Breakfast: pumpkin pie smoothie
Lunch: Paleo spaghetti
Dinner: Roasted chicken with roasted vegetables

Thursday
Breakfast: Fruits
Lunch: avocado slice and and deli meat rollups
Dinner: chicken wrapped in lettuce

Friday
Breakfast: bacon and apples
Lunch: tomato basil chicken
Dinner: slow cooker pork shanks

Saturday
Breakfast: Leftover pork shanks
Lunch: citrus chicken salad stir fry
Dinner: tomato basil mussels

Sunday: Now is the best time to practice the intermittent fasting. It is great for the budget too.

Paleo does not have to be expensive. Enjoy the meals while you save money.

CHAPTER SEVEN:
AMAZING PALEO RECIPES

The great thing about the Paleo diet is you can enjoy a whole course meal and lose weight at the same time. Not to mention, be healthier and even richer (Paleo is not always expensive) in the process. From soups, to appetizers, to main dish, desserts and red wine, Paleo has it all.
Let's get started!!

Paleo Breakfast Recipes

You need a nutritious breakfast to jump start your day. Eating delicious Paleo breakfast can keep you feeling full and satisfied until your next meal. Studies also show that eating breakfast can decrease cravings during the later part of the day and can also boost your energy.

1. Vanilla and Orange Granola

Granola is really simple to make and you can save a lot of time preparing it especially if you have to get out of the house quickly. This granola is perfect for people with sweet tooth. You can also mix it with coconut milk or yogurt if you want.

- 2 cups raw almonds
- 1 cup raw sunflower seeds
- ¼ cup chia seeds
- 2 tbsp orange zest
- ¼ cup olive oil
- 1 cup chopped dried apricots
- 1 cup raw pumpkin seeds
- 1 cup coconut flakes
- 1 tbsp ground vanilla bean
- ½ cup pure maple syrup
- ¼ cup apple butter

Makes 8 servings

Prepare your oven by setting it at 275 degrees. Add almonds to your food processor and blend until it is broken into smaller pieces. Place it in a large bowl. Add the remaining ingredients except for the apricots. Stir well with a spoon and make sure that it is coated. Spread the mixture on top of two baking sheets. Bake for 30 minutes. Stir it three times every 10 minutes. Continue to bake until it is golden brown. Remove it then pour in a bowl. Chop the apricots into very small pieces. Add it to the bowl and stir to coat. Let it cool then store in a container.

Nutrient Facts: 450 calories, 33 g fat, 26 g net carbs, 12 g protein

2. Carrot cake pancakes

These pancakes are made with wholesome ingredients. It uses coconut and almond flour as base. You can also switch the butter with ghee or use your favorite brand. Adjust the sweetness by using applesauce or maple syrup.

- 1 ½ cups almond flour
- ½ cup butter of choice
- 6 eggs
- 1 ½ tsp baking soda
- 2 ½ tsp ginger
- 2/3 cup coconut milk
- 1/3 cup coconut flour
- ½ cup applesauce or agave
- ½ tsp salt
- 2 tbsp cinnamon
- 1 ½ tsp nutmeg
- 2 cups finely shredded carrots

Makes 16 small pancakes

Place all of the ingredients in a large bowl and whisk to combine. The batter should be thick. Heat the pan over medium heat until it reaches about 300 degrees. Coat the pan with the cooking spray. Pour half cup of the batter on the pan. Spread it into a circle and cook for 2 minutes on the first side before flipping it. Cook for one minute on the other side. Feel free to cook it a little bit more if it looks undone. Eat plain or with butter.

Nutrient Facts: 85 calories, 5 g fat, 3.5 g net carbs, 4 g protein

3. Paleo Mexican Chilaquiles

The potato chips absorb the liquid in this dish. This is a great breakfast dish to prepare when you have more time or you want to prepare something special for visitors.

- 2 tbsp ghee
- 2 garlic cloves, minced
- 4 0z diced green chilies
- Half sweet onion, diced
- 1 cup organic chicken broth
- 2 tbsp adobo sauce
- 3 eggs
- 1 cup organic chicken broth
- 2 cups sweet potato chips
- 2 radishes, thinly sliced
- ½ cup salsa
- 2 parsley sprigs, sliced

Makes 2 servings

Set the oven to 375 degrees. Place your pan over medium heat. Use a pan without plastic handle since you will be placing this in your oven. Cook the onion and garlic for a few minutes. Mix in the broth, green chilies and adobo sauce. Stir well to combine. Reduce heat and allow it to simmer. Add the sweet potato chips and stir to coat. Set it aside to let the chips absorb the liquid. You can also add the chips small quantities at a time. Stir one last time to ensure that everything is well coated. Season it with salt and pepper. Break the eggs on top of the mixture. Cook in the oven for 10-14 minutes. It is done when most of the liquid is absorbed. Garnish with the salsa, radish and parsley.

Nutrition facts: 436 calories, 27 g fat, 25 g net carbs, 16 g protein

4. Breakfast Crustless Quiche

This breakfast quiche is creamy and rich in nutrients. Most quiche recipes are heavy in cream and crust. This quiche gets in creaminess from cashews and has a slight smoky flavor from the bacon.

- 1 cup raw cashews
- 4 cups spring greens, loosely packed
- Half lime
- 8 eggs
- 1 cup roasted tomatoes, diced
- ½ tsp salt
- 1/8 tsp garlic powder
- ½ cup water
- 1 tbsp red onion, finely diced
- 1 tbsp olive oil
- 8 slices turkey bacon
- 1 tbsp green chilies, diced
- ½ tsp black pepper

Makes 8 servings

Soak the cashews in a bowl of water at room temperature. Set it aside for 4 hours. Drain the cashews and place it in a blender. Add half cup of fresh water and process the mixture until smooth. Preheat your oven until it reaches 350 degrees. Cook the bacon then crumble into smaller pieces. Set it aside.

Heat olive oil in the pan and cook the onion, spring greens and lime juice. Cook for 3-5 minutes until the green are onions are wilted. Remove it from the heat and dice into small pieces. Mix the bacon, greens, tomatoes, spices, eggs, green chilies and cashew cream in a large bowl. Coat the bake pan with a cooking spray. Pour the batter and spread evenly. Bake for 45 minutes until it is set. Serve with Greek yogurt, avocado or cilantro.

Nutrient facts: 257 calories, 18 g fat, 11 g net carbs, 12 g protein

5. Paleo Cherry Almond Granola

Cherry and almond is a classic combination. This recipe adds coconut, honey and vanilla to make it more delicious.

- 2 cups slivered almonds
- 1 cup sunflower seeds
- ¼ tsp salt
- 4 tbsp honey
- 1 cup cherries, dried
- 1 cup pecans, chopped
- 1 cup unsweetened shredded coconut
- 2 tbsp coconut oil, melted
- 1 tsp vanilla extract

Makes 8 servings

Set the oven at 300 degrees. Mix in the coconut, nuts and salt in a large mixing bowl. Stir to combine. Add the honey, vanilla and coconut oil in a smaller bowl. Whisk to combine then pour over the nut mixture. Spread the mixture on top of a cookie sheet. Bake for 15-20 minutes until it is golden brown. Add in the dried cherries. Stir to combine and allow it cool before serving.

Nutrient facts: 337 calories, 22 g fat, 26 g net carbs, 7 g protein

6. Breakfast Vegetable Frittata

Frittatas are rich in protein so it can keep you full for a longer time. The leeks taste good with the potato crust. It is also easy to make and you can add any vegetable that you have.

- 5 eggs, separated
- 4 small or medium Yukon potatoes, sliced
- 2 small leeks, chopped
- 1 cup kale, chopped
- ½ tsp salt
- ½ tsp black pepper
- 3 tbsp coconut oil
- 8 egg whites
- 2 cloves garlic, minced
- 1 cup tomatoes, chopped
- 1 tbsp fresh basil
- ½ cup shredded cheese

Makes 6 servings

Set the oven at 350 degrees. Add one tablespoon of oil in a pan. Place over medium heat then cook the potatoes one layer at a time. Add more oil if you need to. Cook until it is golden brown. Place on top of a plate lined with paper towel. Add the kale, leek and garlic. Cook for 3 minutes then mix in the tomatoes. Cook for 2 minutes. Remove from heat then set aside. Leave the pan on top of the stove and reduce the heat.

Beat the egg white in a bowl using a mixer until fluffy. Add the egg yolks and whisk for 15 seconds. Place the potatoes on the pan. Layer it carefully to form the crust. Bake for 20 minutes. Turn the broiler for 5 minute and cook until brown.

Nutrient facts: 267 calories, 13 g fat, 21 g net carbs, 15.5 g protein

7. Pear, Turkey and Ginger Patties

These turkey breakfast patties are delicious and easy to prepare. The pears add sweetness to the patties while the ginger adds zest. You can serve this as a simple breakfast or pair it with salad for an elegant brunch.

- 1 ripe pear, chopped
- 1 tsp ginger, grated
- 1 tsp rosemary, minced
- ½ tsp black pepper
- 1 lb ground turkey
- 2 cloves garlic, minced
- 1 tsp sage, minced
- 1 tsp salt
- 2 tbsp coconut oil

Makes 10 patties

Blend the pear in your food processor until it is smooth. Mix in the turkey, garlic, sage, rosemary, garlic, salt and pepper. Stir then scoop the mixture into your hands. Ball it in your palms and flatten it out. Set aside.

Heat the coconut oil in a flat bottom pan. Place the patties on top. Make sure that you leave enough space in between the patties. You can cook the patties in two or three batches. Cook for 4 minutes at the first side until you can easily lift it off the pan. Flip it and cook the other side for 2 minutes. Serve with vegetable.

Nutrient facts: 122 calories, 7 g fat, 2 g net carbs, 12.5 g protein

8. Macadamia waffles

These macadamia waffles are great alternative to pancakes. These waffles are rich in protein and the nuts add healthy oil to the recipe.

- 5 eggs
- ½ cup coconut milk
- 3 tbsp coconut oil, melted
- ¾ tsp baking soda
- ½ tsp salt
- 1 cup raw macadamia nuts
- 3 tbsp honey
- 3 tbsp coconut flour
- ½ tsp vanilla extract
- For the syrup:
- 2 peaches, pitted and sliced
- ½ cup cherries, pitted
- ½ tsp vanilla extract
- 2 plums, pitted and sliced
- ¼ cup honey
- ½ tsp lemon juice

Makes 6 servings

Place the syrup ingredients in a small saucepan. Heat it until it simmers. Keep it at low heat to bring out the flavor of the fruit and make the liquid thick. Prepare the waffles. Preheat the waffle iron. Place all of the ingredients in a blender. Blend for 30 seconds then increase the strength. Blend until the mixture is smooth. Slowly transfer the batter to the waffle iron and spread it evenly with a spoon. Cook the waffle for 45 seconds to one minute. Serve the waffle with the syrup. Serve warm.

Nutrient facts: 421 calories, 31 g fat, 28 g net carbs, 8 g protein

9. Mini Meatloaves with Chipotle and Tomato Relish

Meatloaves are great breakfast options since it is cheap and made with healthy ingredients. However, meatloaves can take too long to cook. You can shorten the cooking time by baking it in muffin tins.

- 1 lb fresh chorizo, casings removed
- 2 tbsp adobo sauce
- ¾ cup almond flour
- 5 cloves garlic, diced
- 1 lb ground beef
- 2 eggs, wild range
- 1 large onion, diced
- Tallow
- For the sauce:
- 1 oz chipotle in adobo sauce
- 2 cups cilantro, chopped
- 1 lime
- 1 pint cherry tomatoes
- 2 tbsp olive oil
- ½ tsp salt
- Half avocado

Makes 18 mini loaves

Set the oven at 350 degrees. Cook the garlic and onion until it is soft. Place half of the onion and garlic mixture in a bowl and the other half in food processor. Place the almond flour, ground beef, adobo sauce, chorizo and egg to the bowl of onion and garlic. Combine the mixture with your hands. Scoop the meatloaf mixture and stuff it into muffin tins. Fill them ¾ full. Place in the oven and bake for 25 minutes until the top is lightly brown.

Cook the tomatoes in the pan until the skin starts to blister. Add the chipotle pepper, salt and olive oil in the food processor. Blend until you have a nice consistency. Pour the sauce into a pan and simmer before adding the cilantro. Garnish with avocado, salt, relish and lime.

Nutrient facts: 210 calories, 14 g fat, 3 g net carbs, 16.7 g protein

10. Cauliflower Breakfast Hash

This is a creamy and spicy Paleo chorizo. The fried eggs add protein and healthy fat to your dish. The flavor comes from the red bell pepper and greens. You can adjust the seasonings to suit your taste.

- 1 lb Paleo chorizo
- 1 onion, chopped
- 2 garlic cloves, chopped
- 6 eggs
- 1 cauliflower head, riced
- 2 tomatoes, chopped
- 1 cup green onions
- ½ cup bell peppers
- Spices of choice
- Oil for frying

Makes 6 servings

Cook the chorizo in a large pan until it is brown. Add in the onions. Stir and cook. Add the garlic and cook for a minute. Add the tomatoes and cauliflower. Fry the mixture for 7 minutes until the rice is cooked and tender. Taste it and adjust the spices if needed. Fry the eggs sunny side up and place on top of your chorizo. Spread the green onions on top then serve.

Nutrition facts: 274 calories, 12 g fat, 10 g net carbs, 30 g protein

Paleo Appetizers

11. Fried Plantain Surprise

http://nourishpaleofoods.files.wordpress.com/
2012/09/apps-and-hash-022.jpg

Ingredients:

- 2 plantains – sliced and squished
- 1 avocado, cubed
- pineapple chunks
- healthy oil
- cilantro leaves

Procedure:
Using the healthy oil, fry the plantain for about 90 seconds on one side and then for another 90 seconds on the other side. Place on a plate. Top with a cubed avocado, followed by a pineapple chunk, a cilantro leaf and then hold them all together using a toothpick.

Nutritional Information:
Bananas and avocado can increase the calorie count but the health benefits of these two are simply worth the calories. Plus, if you are exercising (as you should be when you are in Paleo diet), you would need these two to have that extra energy you need for your strenuous activities. This appetizer could give you around 100-120 calories.

12. Bacon Balls with Mango Honey Mustard Dip

http://paleomg.com/superbowl-snacks-bacon-meatballs-mango-honey-mustard-sauce/

Ingredients:

For the bacon ball
- 1.5 pounds of ground beef (or chicken or pork)
- 6 slices of bacon – cut to smaller pieces of around an inch each
- 1 beaten egg
- ½ onion – diced
- ¼ cup almond flour
- ½ teaspoon chili powder
- sea salt and pepper to taste

Procedure for the bacon ball:
Place the bacon on a skillet and allow it to cook until some fat from the bacon comes out. Add the onion and stir occasionally. Set aside and let it cool. On a large bowl, put the ground beef, the cooled bacon and onion, the flour, egg and the seasonings. Mix thoroughly all the ingredients using your hands. Roll them into a small ball size. You can bake them in the oven for 10-15 minutes or deep-fry them in a skillet.
Ingredients for the dip:

- 1 ripe mango, peeled
- 2 tablespoons of the ground old fashioned mustard
- 1 tablespoon honey
- a pinch of chili powder
- sea salt to taste

Procedure for the dip
Simply put the mango on a blender and let it run for a minute. Add the remaining ingredients. You could adjust the taste by adding more mustard or honey as needed. Pour in a small cup.

Arrange your bacon balls and dip in a plate. Provide toothpicks on the bacon balls for the guests to use.

Nutritional information:
You can consume a total of around 400 calories for every 5 bacon balls dipped in the mango honey mustard sauce. That amount is actually too much and heavy for your stomach. Try to limit to 1-2 of this bacon ball per meal. That way, you can have enough space for other dishes and your calories would not be that high after the meal.

Paleo Lunch Recipes

Taking a break from work can help you relieve stress and collect your thoughts. Prepare these delicious and healthy lunches to keep you satiated and full.

13. Gluten Free and Dairy Free Chicken Tortilla Soup

http://eatdrinkpaleo.com.au/wp-content/uploads/2012/09/gazpacho_paleo.jpg

Ingredients:
- 2 large chicken breasts cut into ½ inch strips. Remove all skins.
- 800 grams diced tomatoes
- 900 ml or 32 ounces organic chicken broth
- 1 diced onion
- 2 diced and de-seeded jalapenos
- 2 cups carrots – shredded
- 2 cups chopped celery
- 4 cloves of minced garlic
- 2 tablespoons tomato paste
- 1 teaspoon chili powder
- sea salt to taste
- ½ teaspoon cracked pepper
- 1 tablespoon olive oil
- 1-2 cups water
- 1/3 cup cilantro – chopped fine
- avocado slice - optional

Procedure:
In a large pot, pour ¼ cup chicken broth and a dash of olive oil. Place the pot over medium high heat. Add the onions, garlic and jalapeno and cook until soft. Add more broth as needed plus the sea salt and cracked pepper. Then add all the remaining ingredients except for the cilantro and avocado

slices. Cover and cook on low heat for 2 hours. Shred the cooked chicken. Top with avocado slice and fresh cilantro. Serve hot!

Nutritional Information: 1 serving
The estimated calorie count for chicken tortilla soup is at 140 per serving.Do not forget to remove all chicken skins as this will cause additional 50 calories if the skins are left intact. This meal is rich in proteins (8.0 grams). It is also a good source of the electrolyte Potassium at 780 mg. Total carbohydrate is at 22.0 mg. Make sure that you use all Paleo allowed ingredients only as calorie count would be different otherwise.

Here is another soup that would "warm" the heart of your special ones.

14. Mojo Avocado Chicken Cups

This Cuban inspired dish is a great way to use your leftover chicken in avocado cups. These are delicious and quick lunch recipes that can be paired with simple salad.

- 1 tbsp coconut oil
- ¼ cup orange juice
- ½ tsp oregano leaves, dried
- ½ onion, finely chopped
- 1 mango, chopped into bite size
- 1 tbsp lime juice
- 3 garlic cloves, minced
- ¼ cup lemon juice
- ½ lb chicken, shredded or chopped
- 2 avocados, medium, cut in half with the pits removed
- ¼ cup cilantro leaves, chopped
- ½ tsp salt

Makes 3 servings

Add the oil to the pan and cook the garlic. Stir and cook until it is soft and translucent. Pour the lemon juice to the pan. To make the sauce, add the oregano leaves. Increase the heat and bring to a simmer. Pour the mojo in a bowl and set it aside.

Add ½ tbsp oil in a pan (the rest would be used later). Cook the shredded chicken until done. Add the sliced onion and 4 tablespoon mojo sauce. Toss the mixture to coat. Reduce the heat and cook for another 6 minutes until the onions become soft. Pour the remaining sauce then remove from the heat.

Cut the skin from the avocado's rounded end to prevent it from rolling when placed on plates. Place the chicken on top and add the mango, lime, salt, and cilantro. Serve.

Nutrient facts: 454 calories, 33 g fat, 8 g net carbs, 25 g protein

15. Apple Braised Pork Shank

Pork shanks are inexpensive but it is full of flavor when braised. It is also rich in glycerin and is very easy to prepare.

- 4 lb pork shank
- 4 apples
- ½ head Napa cabbage
- 1 bay leaf
- 1 tsp ginger, grated
- 1 whole mace avril
- 1 orange zest
- 1 large onion
- 3 tbsp coconut oil
- 1 cup white wine
- ½ tsp whole cloves
- 1 stick cinnamon

Makes 8 servings

Set your oven at 300 degrees. Peel and remove the core of the apple. Chop each apple to 8-10 pieces. Cut the onion into large wedges. Chop the Napa cabbage. Heat the oil in a Dutch oven over medium heat. Cook the shank in several batches. Cook for 3 minutes at each side. Add more lard if desired.

Add onion to your pot and cook until it is brown. Mix in the cabbage, apple, orange zest, juice, wine and spices to the pot. Stir then add the shanks. Bake in the oven for 3 hours.

Make the gravy. Set the shanks aside and discard the bay leaf, mace and cinnamon. Blend the mixture until smooth. You can simmer the mixture to make it thicker. Serve with the meat.

Nutrient facts: 411 calories, 23 g fat, 16 g net carbs, 29 g protein

16. Paleo Plantain Curry Lasagna

This is a combination of classic curry flavor in a Puerto Rican dish. The plantain and egg are used instead of noodles.

- 6 ripe plantains
- 8 eggs
- 2 tbsp red palm oil
- 1 yellow onion, medium
- 6 cloves garlic, diced
- 4 tsp turmeric
- 3 tsp coriander
- 1 tsp cardamom
- ½ tsp pepper
- ½ tsp caraway seeds
- 4 tbsp coconut oil
- 2 lb ground beef
- 1 carrot
- 1 celery stalks
- 2 tsp salt
- 2 tsp cumin
- 2 tsp ground ginger
- ½ tsp cinnamon
- ½ tsp anise
- ½ can coconut milk

Makes 10 servings

Cut the plantains crosswise and peel it. Cut it into quarter of an inch slices. Heat the coconut oil in a pan. Fry the slices for 3 minutes on each side until brown. Set this aside. Dice the carrot, celery and onion. You can also mix all of your spices in a bowl. Set the oven at 350 degrees. Heat the red palm oil over medium heat. Mix in the celery, onion and carrot. Cook until it is fragrant and brown.

Add the beef and stir frequently for 8 minutes. Add the seasonings and coconut milk. Simmer and continue to cook for 15 minutes. You can add more milk if it looks too dry. It should be thick and creamy.

Assemble the lasagna. Whisk the eggs in a bowl and pour half at the bottom of a dish. Cook in the oven for 7 minutes. Layer half of the plantain slices on top of the egg. Pour the meat sauce on top. Place another layer of plantain slice on top. Whisk the eggs and pour on top of the lasagna. Bake for 30-35 minutes. Allow to cool before serving.

Nutrient facts: 441 calories, 18 g fat, 33 g net carbs, 34 g protein

17. Pomegranate Molasses Glazed Salmon

Pomegranate molasses is a common ingredient in Lebanese cooking. It is made by simmering the juice of the fruit until thick. It is deliciously paired with the salmon.

- 4 salmon fillets
- 4 garlic cloves, crushed
- 2 tbsp pomegranate molasses
- 1 tbsp ginger, grated
- ¼ cup orange juice
- 1 tbsp coconut oil

Makes 4 servings

Mix the orange juice, ginger and garlic in a bowl. Add 2 tablespoon of the molasses and pour it over the salmon. Let it marinate for 15 minutes. Set the oven at 425 degrees. Cover the baking sheet with foil. Grease it with coconut oil. You can skip this step if your salmon has skin. Place the fish on the baking sheet then spread more molasses on each salmon. Bake for 12-15 minutes until it looks opaque.

Nutrient facts: 310 calories, 14.5 g fat, 11 g net carbs, 35 g protein

18. Chicken Vegetable Soup

http://paleoonabudget.com/wp-content/
uploads/2014/01/Paleo_Chicken_Vegetable_Soup-3.jpg

Ingredients:
- 2-4 cups shredded chicken (boiled)
- 1 tablespoon healthy oil of your choice
- 1 onion- diced
- 3 carrots – diced
- 1 zucchini – diced
- ¼ butternut aquash –cubed
- 12 ounces mushroom – diced
- 1 teaspoon each of rosemary, basil and dried thyme
- 1 tablespoon apple cider vinegar
- sea salt and pepper to taste
- 500 ml chicken broth
- lemon – optional

Procedure:
In a large pot, put all your vegetables, chicken, oil, and stir occasionally. Add the remaining ingredients together with the chicken broth and cook slowly for an hour. Before you serve, you can squeeze one lemon (optional) to make it more delicious. Serve immediately.

Nutritional information:
Total calorie count would be estimated at 150. With much vegetable as ingredients, the dietary fiber is at 12% of % daily value.

19. Paleo Steak and Kidney Pie

This is a delicious pie recipe with a light and rich crust that resembles a pudding.

- 3 lb steak
- 6 oz Portobello mushrooms
- 1 bay leaf
- ½ tsp salt
- 3 carrots, medium
- 2 tbsp arrowroot powder
- 1 ½ lb lamb kidney
- 1 large sweet onion
- ½ tbsp fish sauce
- ½ tsp pepper, to taste
- 2 cups beef stock
- 4 tbsp bacon grease
- For the pastry:
- 1 cup coconut milk
- 1/3 cup tapioca starch
- 4 eggs
- ½ cup palm shortening
- 1/3 cup coconut flour
- 1/3 cup arrowroot powder
- ½ tsp salt

Makes 10 servings

Slice the kidney and steak into thick slices. Cut the carrots into thick rounds. Slice the mushrooms in half and chop the onion into half moons. Heat the bacon grease in a large pan. Brown the kidney and meat and set aside. Add more bacon grease to the pan and cook the onion slices for 5 minutes. Add the mushrooms and carrots. Cook for 3 minutes. Return the meat to the pot and add the arrowroot powder. Season it with bay leaf and fish sauce. Simmer and adjust the seasoning if desired. Pour in a large casserole and let it cool to room temperature.

64

Mix the salt and flour. Crack the eggs in a separate bowl. Set the oven at 425 degrees. Heat the shortening and milk until it simmers. Pour on top of the flour quickly. Add the eggs one at a time and stir to combine. You should have thick and sticky dough. Pour the dough on top of the steak and kidney mixture. Spread evenly then bake for 25 minutes.

Nutrient facts: 516 calories, 20 g fat, 14 g net carbohydrates, 63.5 g protein

20. Asian Inspired Chicken Wings

This is inspired by traditional Chinese cuisine. It has a distinct Asian flavor but it can be paired with any side dish.

- 3 lb chicken wings, separated
- 4 garlic cloves, chopped
- 1 tsp anise seed
- ½ cup coconut aminos
- 2 tbsp coconut vinegar
- 2 tbsp sesame oil
- 2 tbsp coconut oil
- 1 tbsp ginger, chopped
- 1 tsp fennel seed
- 2 tbsp honey
- 1 tbsp fish sauce

Makes 6 servings

Place the chicken wings in a bowl. Heat the oil in a saucepan. Add the fennel, ginger, anise and garlic. Stir until it is fragrant. Add the vinegar, honey, fish sauce and coconut aminos. Boil and simmer for one minute. Add the sesame oil. Pour the mixture over the chicken wings and stir to coat. Marinate for 24 hours. Drain and cook the wings in a grill. Turn once to cook the other side. You can also bake it for 45 minutes at 375 degrees.

Nutrient facts: 541 calories, 26 g fat, 8 g net carbohydrates, 66 g protein

21. Parchment Salmon With Herb

Herbs add natural flavor to your dish without the excess chemicals and preservatives. You can make a large batch of herbs and store it in a container so that you can quickly prepare this dish.

- 1 cup unsalted butter, softened
- 4 garlic cloves, crushed
- 1/3 cup parsley
- ¼ tsp ground pepper, to taste
- 1 lemon, zest
- ½ cup dill
- ½ tsp salt
- 4 8oz salmon fillet

Makes 4 servings

Mix the herbs and lemon zest in the food processor and blend until it is fine. Add the herb mixture to a bowl and stir to combine. Set the oven at 350 degrees. Lay a sheet of tin foil on a baking sheet. The foil should be twice as long as the fish fillet. Place the fish on the foil and make sure to leave enough space between the fish. Scoop the herb and spread it on top of the fillet. Spread one tablespoon of water around the fish. Bake this for 20 minutes until the fish is opaque.

Nutrient facts: 668 calories, 57 g fat, 4.5 g net carbs, 36.7 g protein

22. Paleo Spaghetti and Meatballs

This Paleo spaghetti version is made with squash for pasta. The secret to this delicious dish is the use of fresh spices. It might seem that you are using too much oregano and basil but they are needed to bring out the flavor.

- 3 lb summer squash
- 16 garlic cloves, minced
- 1 ½ cups whole black olive
- ¾ cup basil, chopped
- 1 tbsp salt
- 10 oz mushrooms, sliced
- 5 slices bacon
- For the meatballs:
- ¼ tsp salt
- 2 lb ground beef
- ¼ cup oregano, chopped

Makes 6 servings

Use a vegetable spiraler to cut your squash into noodles. Place in a strainer and season it with salt. Let it sit for an hour. Rinse though with water. Let the noodles drain and set it on top of paper towels to absorb the water.

Chop the bacon into small pieces. Place a large pan or pot over medium heat. Cook the bacon until it is brown. Mix in the garlic and mushrooms. Continue to cook for 8 minutes until the mushrooms are soft and brown. Add the squash noodles and olives. Toss and stir for 5 minutes until it is cooked. Add the basil and stir for a few seconds. Add the meatballs and serve.

Nutrient facts: 280 calories, 12.6 g fat, 11 g net carbs, 51 g protein

23. Chicken Burgers with Maple Syrup

The strong flavor of maple syrup is compatible with the cranberries. This dish has the perfect blend of sweet and savory.

- 2 ½ lb ground chicken or turkey
- 1 large apple
- 2 tsp rosemary, chopped
- 8 oz bacon
- 1 onion
- ½ tsp salt
- For the sauce:
- ½ cup maple syrup
- 2 cups frozen cranberries
- ¼ cup water

Makes 10 servings

Place the bacon in the pan and cook until it is crispy. Dice the onion and apple. Chop the rosemary. Remove the bacon from the pan and add the fat and onion. Cook for 5 minutes until the onions are soft. Add the rosemary and apple. Continue to cook until it is done.

Chop the bacon into slices. Combine the chicken, onion mix, apple and bacon. Mix with your hands and form into patties. Add fat to a pan and cook the patties. Flip once and cook for one minute.

Make the sauce. Combine the ingredients in a saucepan and boil. Simmer for 10 minutes and stir occasionally. Serve with the burgers.

Nutrient facts: 406 calories, 18 g fat, 15 g net carbs, 42 g protein

24. Paleo Chicken Pad Thai

This is a Paleo vesion of an ethnic food. The broccoli and carrots replace the pasta noodles and they also add more nutritional value to your dish. This recipe also makes use of a lot of spices to bring out its flavor.

- 1 ½ lb chicken, cut into chunks
- 5 garlic cloves, chopped
- 1 tbsp coconut aminos
- ½ tbsp coconut vinegar
- 5 green onion, chopped
- 2 medium carrots, julienned
- 5 tbsp extra virgin coconut oil
- 3 tbsp fish sauce
- 4 tbsp lime juice
- 5 tbsp cilantro, chopped
- 12 oz broccoli slaw

Makes 6 servings

Place a large pan over medium heat. Add in the garlic and onion. Stir and cook for a minute. Place the chicken on the pan and cook for 3-5 minutes. Make sure to stir it frequently until it is golden brown. Mix in the vinegar, fish sauce, coconut aminos and lime juice. Cook and simmer until it is cooked through. Add the carrots and broccoli. Cook until it is soft but still firm. Toss to coat then garnish the dish with cilantro and green onions.

Nutrient facts: 326 calories, 15 g fat, 8 g net carbs, 35.6 g protein

Paleo Dinner Recipes

Dinner is often the most favored meal of the day since it is the time where you can reward your hard work with delicious food. These recipes are great comfort foods and are also perfect for special occasions.

25. Paleo Strip Steak with Cucumber Salad
http://paleoleap.com/steak-cucumber-salad/

Ingredients:
- 1 1/2 pounds of your favorite steak (sirloin steak is recommended)
- 1 cucumber- sliced
- 2 cloves minced garlic
- 1 tablespoon coconut oil
- ¼ cup water
- 2 fresh lime juice
- 1 tablespoon fresh chives – minced
- sea salt and pepper to taste

Procedure:
Season the steak by putting sea salt and pepper and let it stand for 15 minutes. While waiting for that, sauté the garlic with the coconut oil.Add the lime juice, water and season with seal salt and pepper. Allow to boil and then remove from heat after two minutes. Set aside and let it cool.

Grill the steaks until the desired doneness. Cut into strips. Place the sliced cucumber on a plate and top with the steaks and sauce.

This dish is healthy, delicious and filling. You do not need a large amount to feel satiated.

Nutritional Information:
One small serving of steak is around 150 calories. Try to limit your intake of the strip steaks into maximum of three pieces.

Another mouth watering main dish
If you are more inclined on fish, maybe you would prefer this recipe instead for your main dish. This is called Paleo Red Snapper Curry with vegetables.

For this recipe however, the vegetables used were ginger, carrots and broccoli. You could always mix and match the vegetables of your choice.

26. Veal, Carrot and Chestnut Ragout

Chestnuts add a sweet flavor to dishes especially stews. Chestnuts are often paired with veal in many Italian cuisines. Try to use fresh chestnuts as much as possible to bring out the flavor.

- 18 fresh chestnuts
- 2 ½ lb veal cut into small piece
- 1 ½ cups onion, chopped
- 1 bay leaf
- ¾ cup dry white wine
- 3 tbsp fresh sage, chopped
- 4 tbsp olive oil
- 1 ½ tbsp garlic, chopped
- 2 1/2 cups low salt chicken broth
- 6 medium carrots, peeled and cut into small pieces

Makes 8 servings

Set the oven at 400 degrees. Use a knife to cut X in each of the chestnuts. Place it in a pan. Bake until the shells are loose and it is soft. This usually takes about 30 minutes. Let it cool then remove the shell. Set aside.

Pat the meat pieces with paper towels. Season it with pepper. Add oil in a large pan and cook the veal until it is brown on all the sides. This will take about 10 minutes. Remove from pan and place in a large bowl.

Heat the oil in the same pot. Add in the bay leaf, onion and garlic. Simmer and cook until it is tender. Make sure to stir continuously. Stir in the wine and broth. Add veal and juice from the bowl. Boil then simmer for 45 minutes while stirring constantly. Add the carrots to the stew and cook until it is tender. The liquid should be reduced to a thick consistency. Simmer for 3 minutes and remove the bay leaf. Transfer to a bowl.

Nutrient facts: 480 calories, 18 g fat, 32 g net carbs, 37 g protein

27. Japanese Whitefish and Noodle Soup

This dish is a great way to add seaweed into your diet. Seaweed is rich in iodine and other nutrients. This soup is based on Japanese Dashi with the noodles replaced by kelp noodles. You can also add other seafood like shrimp, squid and scallops.

- 2 pieces kombu kelp
- 4 cups water
- 1 lb kelp noodles
- 1 tbsp coconut water vinegar
- 1 cup lightly packed bonito flakes
- 2 tilapia or cod
- 2 tbsp coconut aminos
- 4 cups loosely packed greens

Makes 3 servings

Place the bonito and kombu in a large pot and add water. Bring to a boil then reduce the temperature and simmer for 10 minutes. Chop the greens and place in a bowl. Cut fish into cubes. Rinse the kelp in running water. Strain the broth using a cheese cloth to remove the kombu and bonito. Return the broth to the pot. Mix in the coconut vinegar and coconut aminos. Add the fish to the pot and cook until done. If you are using tough greens like snow peas, cabbage and bok choy, add it at the same time as the fish but if you are using tender greens like chard and spinach add them after the fish is cooked. Mix in the kelp noodles. Simmer for 3 minutes before serving.

Nutrient facts: 105 calories, 0.7 g fat, 1.3 g net carbs, 18 g protein

28. Tourtiere Shepherd's Pie

Tourtiere is a French Canadian meat pie that is usually made with ground pork. This recipe uses a combination of pork and grass fed bison. This is a deliciously comforting dish perfect for cold nights.

For the base:
- 4 lb ground meat
- 6 celery stalks, chopped
- 4 bay leaves
- 1/3 cup arrowroot powder
- 2 medium onion, chopped
- 3 tbsp rosemary sprig
- 8 oz mushroom, chopped
- 1 tsp salt to taste
- For the top:
- 2 tbsp grass fed butter
- ½ tsp salt to taste
- 1 ½ heads of cauliflower
- 1 tsp garlic powder

Makes 8 servings

Place a large pot over medium heat. Cook the meat then add the bay leaves, celery, onions and rosemary. Cook until the meat is brown. Do not drain the fat. Add in the mushrooms and cook until the celery and mushrooms are tender. Stir the mixture occasionally until the meat is cooked. Season it with salt to taste. Add in the arrowroot powder and cook for 3 minutes. Remove from heat. Discard the bay leaves and rosemary. Pour the mixture into a deep pan. Spread evenly using a spoon or spatula.

Steam the cauliflower in a pot with salted water. Cook until it is very tender. Drain the cauliflower and return it to the pot. Process it in a blender or mash with a potato masher. Add the cooking fat, salt and garlic powder. Stir well to combine. Spread the cauliflower mixture on top of the meat. Bake for

40 minutes at 375 degrees until the top is brown. Cool for 10 minutes before serving.

Nutrient facts: 629 calories, 37.5 g fat, 10.5 g net carbs, 57 g protein

29. Pork Chow Mein

This is a delicious and easy to prepare dinner. Make sure to slice the meat and vegetable thinly for this dish to make it tastier. The kelp noodles also add flavor and texture to this dish.

- 2 tbsp coconut oil
- 1 small onion, sliced in wedges
- 5 oz can bamboo shoots, sliced
- 8 baby mushrooms
- 1 cup bone broth
- 1 lb kelp noodles
- 1 lb pork loin chops, sliced thinly
- 5 oz can water chestnuts, sliced
- 4 dried shiitake mushrooms
- 3 baby bok choy
- 1 tbsp coconut vinegar
- 1 green onion

Makes 5 servings
Soak the dried mushrooms in water and set aside for half an hour. Rinse the mushrooms and slice it into thin strips. Slice the onion in wedges. Chop the mushrooms in quarters and separate the leaves of bok choy. Drain and rinse the chestnuts and bamboo shoots. Rinse the kelp noodles in flowing water.

Heat a large pan and add the coconut oil. Cook the pork and stir frequently until the meat is brown. Add the mushrooms, onion and bok choy. Slowly pour the coconut vinegar and broth. Cook and stir frequently for 10 minutes until the pork is done but the vegetables are al dente. Increase the heat. Create a hole in the middle by pushing the pork and vegetable to the sides. Place the kelp noodles in the middle and simmer for 3 minutes. Break the kelp noodles and spread it to the chow mein. Garnish with green onions before serving.

Nutrient facts: 488 calories, 29 g fat, 19 g net carbs, 34 g protein

30. Pumpkin chili

This is a great recipe to try if you have a lot of pumpkin. This pumpkin chili is flavorful and has a slightly sweet taste that is reminiscent of curry. This dish is also rich in nutrients and low in carbohydrates.

- 1 medium pumpkin, peeled and cut into cubes
- 2 tbsp coconut oil, melted
- 1 lb ground beef
- 8 celery stalks, chopped
- 3 bay laves
- 1 ½ tbsp cumin
- 1 tsp nutmeg
- ¼ tsp cayenne
- 1 ½ tbsp oregano, chopped
- 1 bunch fresh spinach, chopped
- 6 oz tomato paste
- ½ tsp salt to taste
- 1 large sweet potato, peeled and cubed
- 2 lb ground turkey
- 2 onions, chopped
- 8 garlic cloves, chopped
- 3 tbsp chili powder to taste
- 1 tsp cinnamon
- 2 tsp cocoa powder
- 1 ½ tbsp basil, chopped
- 2 tbsp cilantro, chopped
- 3 can diced tomatoes
- 2 cups pumpkin puree

Makes 10 servings

Combine the sweet potato and pumpkin in a bowl. Add the oil and toss to combine. Spread it evenly in a baking pan and bake for 30 minutes at 350 degrees until it is brown and soft. Cook the beef and turkey in a pan. Add the bay leaves, onion, celery and garlic in a pot. Stir gently to avoid breaking the meat into very small pieces. Add the cocoa, nutmeg, chili, cumin and cinnamon once the meat is cooked. Cook and stir until soft and fragrant. Add the tomato paste, puree, tomatoes and salt. Simmer and reduce the heat. Simmer for 15 minutes until the celery is soft. Garnish with spinach, oregano and basil. Add the sweet potato and pumpkin. Stir to combine.

Nutrient facts: 384 calories, 17 g fat, 15 g net carbs, 43 g protein

31. Red Curry Snapper & Ginger Honey Carrots

http://eatdrinkpaleo.com.au/20-minute-paleo-meals-red-curry-snapper-ginger-honey-carrots-recipe/

The beauty of this recipe is you can whip this within 20 minutes. Here is how you can do this.

Ingredients:
- 2 red snapper. Remove the skins.
- 1 teaspoon curry paste
- ½ teaspoon sea salt
- 2 tablespoons virgin olive oil
- 10 baby carrots (boiled, peeled and cut into halves)
- 2 cups broccoli
- 1 garlic clove
- ½ tablespoon fresh ginger – thinly sliced
- 1 tablespoon lemon juice
- 1 teaspoon honey
- 1 tablespoon fish sauce
- drizzle of lime or lemon

Procedure:
Mix the curry paste, olive oil and sea salt. Brush the red snappers with the mixture. Set aside for 15 minutes for the taste to set in.

Heat the coconut oil in a skillet. Add the ginger and the carrots (already boiled, peeled and cut into two) and cook for 2 minutes. Add the rest of the ingredients except for the fish and broccoli. When the ginger and the baby carrots seem to be caramelized, add the olive oil and fry the fish fillet. Cook for around 3 minutes on each side. Add the blanched broccoli.

Before you serve, you may want to add a drizzle of lemon or lime to give that zesty taste.

Nutritional Information:
A single serving of red snapper is equivalent to 200-250 calories. That's why you can afford to have another serving if you wish.

32. Meatballs with Cacik

Cacik is a Turkish dish that originally made with mint, yogurt and cucumber. The best thing about this recipe is that it can be made ahead of time. The longer the meat is marinated with the seasoning, the better it tastes. This recipe also includes organ meat but you can hardly notice it because of the seasonings.

- 2 lb ground meat
- 6 cloves garlic, crushed
- 1 ½ tsp chili powder
- 1 tsp paprika
- 1 cup flaxseed meal
- 2 tbsp extra virgin coconut oil
- ¾ cups parsley, chopped
- 1 tbsp cumin seed, ground
- ¾ tsp salt to taste
- ½ tsp pepper
- 1 large onion, diced
- For the cacik:
- 1 cup coconut milk yogurt
- 4 garlic cloves, crushed
- 3 tbsp extra virgin olive oil
- 1 ½ cucumbers
- 2 tsp salt
- 2 tbsp mint, chopped

Makes 10 servings

Combine the ground meat and the seasoning in a bowl. Place in the refrigerator for an hour to marinate. Heat the coconut oil in a large pan over medium heat. Cook the diced onion and cook until soft. Remove and let it cool. Set the oven at 400 degrees. Cover the baking sheet with parchment paper. Combine the onion and flaxseed meal to the meat. Scoop the meat into your hands to make the meatballs. Place on top of the baking sheet. Bake for 20 minutes.

Make the cacik. Slice the cucumbers thinly and season with salt. Let it soak for 1 hour. Rinse the cucumber and place it on top of paper towels. Combine the mint, cucumber, yogurt and garlic in a bowl. Refrigerate for 1-8 hours. Stir in the olive oil and serve with meatballs.

Nutrient facts: 377 calories, 25 g fat, 5 g net carbs, 25 g protein

33. Chicken Puttanesca

The traditional puttanesca sauce is made from whorish sauce of tomatoes, capers, garlic, anchovies and chili. This dish can cook quickly so you have to prepare all of the ingredients beforehand.

- ¼ cup extra virgin olive oil, divided
- 4 garlic cloves, minced
- ½ cup Italian olives, pitted and chopped
- 4 boneless anchovy fillet, chopped
- 1 lb assorted fresh tomatoes, diced
- 4 boneless chicken breasts
- 1 small red onion, diced
- 1 tbsp capers, drained and chopped
- ½ tsp crushed red chili flakes
- Salt and pepper to taste

Makes 4 servings

Set the oven to 450 degrees. Set a pan over medium heat. Coat the chicken with oil and season with salt and pepper. Cook in the pan until one side is golden brown. Flip the chicken and place the pan into the oven. Roast for 8 minutes. Once it is firm, remove and place the pan on top of the stove. Remove the chicken breast and transfer to plates. Add the olives, capers, anchovies, oil, garlic, chili and onion. Stir the ingredients for a minute. Add the tomatoes and adjust the seasoning. Cook the sauce until it is thick. Pour over the chicken before serving.

Nutrient facts: 386 calories, 20 g fat, 7 g net carbs, 38 g protein

34. West Coast Casserole

This dish is inspired by beef sandwiches that are made with cheese, sauerkraut and corned beef. This Paleo version has the same taste and texture but without the grains.

- 2 tbsp lard
- 4 garlic clove, minced
- ½ tsp cinnamon, ground
- ¼ tsp allspice, ground
- 2 lb ground beef
- ½ cup sour cream
- 1 tsp caraway seeds, whole
- Salt and pepper to taste
- 1 medium onion, diced
- 2 bay leaves
- ¼ tsp cloves, ground
- ¼ tsp dried juniper berries
- ½ cup Dijon mustard
- 1 lb sauerkraut, drained
- ½ lb Swiss cheese, grated

Makes 6 servings

Set the oven to 350 degrees. Place a large pan over medium heat and melt the butter. Add the garlic and onion. Cook until it is translucent. Add the allspice, bay leaves, cinnamon, berries, cloves, salt and pepper. Cook for a few minutes then add the beef. Adjust the taste if needed. Break the ground beef and strain excess liquid. Scoop the ground meat at the bottom of the casserole pan. Mix the sour cream and mustard in a bowl. Stir then pour over the beef. Squeeze the sauerkraut to remove excess moisture. Spread on top of the beef and mustard. Sprinkle with caraway seeds. Spread the Swiss cheese on top and bake for 30 minutes until the cheese is brown and melted. Allow to rest before serving.

Nutrient facts: 644 calories, 49 g fat, 7.5 g net carbs, 38 g protein

35. Skinny Buffalo Chicken Strips

This chicken dish is spicy and flavorful. It is also low in fat and sodium.

- 2 lb boneless and skinless chicken breast
- ½ cup water
- 2 tbsp dried oregano
- 2 tbsp ground cumin
- ½ cup cider vinegar
- 3 tbsp cayenne pepper
- 2 tbsp garlic powder
- 2 tbsp chili powder

Makes 6 servings

Cut the chicken into strips. Place the chicken in a sealable bag and mix in the water, pepper and vinegar. Rub the spices into the chicken. Make sure that cayenne is distributed evenly. Set the oven at 350 degrees. Place the chicken on the baking sheet. Sprinkle with the seasonings and bake for 20 minutes until done.

Nutrient facts: 2014 calories, 3.5 g fat, 4.3 g net carbs, 36 g protein

36. Ginger Steak Salad

This is a quick and easy dinner recipe that is full of flavors and high in protein. The vegetables also add nutritional value to the dish.

- 2 tbsp coconut oil, divided
- 1 tsp turmeric, ground
- 1 tsp cumin seed, ground
- 4 cups baby spinach, washed and stems removed
- 420 g cauliflower, cut into florets
- 1 ½ lb beef flank, cut into portions
- ½ cup sweet and spicy tomato jam
- Salt and pepper to taste

Makes 4 servings

Set your oven to 400 degrees. Toss the cauliflower in a bowl of oil, turmeric, salt and pepper. Place the cauliflower in a baking sheet and roast for 12 minutes. Set the pan on top of medium heat. Season the beef with pepper, cumin and salt. Add oil to the pan and cook the beef for 5 minutes on each side. Combine the spinach, tomato jam, salt and pepper. Add the cauliflower to the bowl and toss to coat. Divide evenly into 4 plates. Slice the steak into strips and add to the salad.

Nutrient facts: 552 calories, 37 g fat, 8 g net carbs, 15 g protein

Paleo Dessert Recipes

A healthy dessert is a great way to end your meal. Just because you cannot use some ingredients does not mean that you have to sacrifice delicious dessert.

37. Paleo banana strawberry sorbet

https://static.squarespace.com/static/52fd86dfe4b0a44284e8af84/53220664e4b0839c3a2ca432/532206f7e4b0839c3a2cccad/1394738935622/1000w/

Ingredients:
- 1 ripe banana
- 2 cups fresh strawberries
- ½ cup coconut cream
- 1 teaspoon agave nectar

Procedure:
Simply combine all ingredients and blend. Place in the freezer and take it out when it is solid but not completely frozen. Scoop it out and place in a glass. Place a fresh strawberry as an edible decoration and there you have it!

Nutritional Information:
This yummy dessert would only cause you around 30-35 calories per small glass. And the calories are totally worth it!

38. Pumpkin Cake Cookies

Treat yourself to delicious cookies sweetened with natural spices and honey. These Paleo cookies are great to have during the Holidays so you won't be tempted to binge on sugary desserts.

- ¾ cup pumpkin puree
- 5 eggs
- 2 tbsp honey
- ½ tsp baking power
- ½ tsp nutmeg
- 1 cup dark chocolate chips
- ¼ cup coconut oil, melted
- 1 tsp vanilla extract
- 1/3 cup coconut flour
- 1 tsp cinnamon
- ¼ tsp ground cloves

Makes 15 cookies

Set your oven to 375 degrees. Combine the puree, eggs, honey, oil and vanilla in a large bowl. Whisk the ingredients to combine. In a separate bowl, add the baking powder, coconut flour and spices. Add the spices to the pumpkin mixture. Stir until the mixture is free of lumps. Add the chocolate chips. Line the baking sheet with parchment paper. Scoop 2 tablespoon of dough and drop on the baking sheet. Flatten and then bake for 10 minutes until done. Allow it to cool for 10 minutes before serving.

Nutrient facts: 115 calories, 7.6 g fat, 9 g net carbs, 3 g protein

39. Spinach Brownies

Children are notorious for avoiding vegetables. Adding greens to their chocolate dessert is a good way to increase the nutrient content of the brownies without compromising the taste.

- 1 ¼ cups frozen spinach, chopped
- 6 oz semisweet chocolate
- ½ cup palm shortening
- 1 tbsp honey
- ½ cup cocoa powder
- ¼ tsp baking soda
- ½ tsp cream of tartar
- 1 cup pureed green plantain
- ½ cup extra virgin coconut oil
- 6 eggs
- 1 tbsp molasses
- 1 tbsp vanilla
- ½ tsp salt
- ½ tsp cinnamon

Makes 24 brownies

Set the oven at 325 degrees. Cover the baking pan with wax paper. Place a small saucepan on top of a stove then melt the chocolate and coconut oil. Mix in the vanilla and stir to incorporate. Let it cool. Combine the cream of tartar, baking soda, cinnamon, salt and cocoa powder. Whisk to combine. Place the honey, spinach, egg, molasses and plantain in the food processor. Blend until the mixture is smooth. Add the palm shortening and blend well until everything is incorporated.

Add the chocolate to the egg mixture and continue the blending process. Add the dry ingredients and stir to combine. Pour the batter to the pan. Spread the mixture using a spoon or spatula. Bake for 40 minutes. Let it cool then cut into squares.

Nutrient facts: 112 calories, 8 g fat, 8 g net carbs, 2 g protein

40. Sticky Date Cupcakes

These cupcakes are quick and easy to make. It has a thick date ganache that adds sweetness to the cupcakes.

Grass fed butter for greasing

- 12 dates
- 3 tbsp coconut flour
- 2 eggs
- ½ tsp baking powder
- 10 tbsp water
- 1 ½ ripe banana, peeled and chopped
- 1 tbsp vanilla extract
- 1tsp honey

For the date ganache:

- ½ orange, juiced
- 1 tsp vanilla extract
- Fresh raspberries for garnish
- 5 dates, chopped
- 3 tbsp almond milk
- 1 tsp honey

Makes 5 servings

Set the oven at 185 degrees. Grease your muffin tins with grass fed butter. Set aside. Place dates and water in a saucepan. Simmer over low heat until it breaks down and thickens. Mash the mixture using a fork. Place banana, baking powder, vanilla, flour and egg in a blender. Process until combined. Add the dates to the banana. Stir to combine. Scoop it into the ramekins. Bake for 20 minutes.

Combine the ganache ingredients in a pot. Simmer for 4 minutes until the dates are tender. Mash with fork and whisk. Let the muffins cool before spreading the ganache on top. Add a few raspberries for garnish.

Nutrient facts: 203 calories, 4.5 g fat, 30 g net carbs, 4.2 g protein

41. Apple Cinnamon Coffee Cake
with Walnut Topping

This is a Paleo version of a coffee cake. The crunch top pairs great with the chewy cake.

- ½ cup almond flour
- 2 tbsp coconut flour
- 1 tbsp cinnamon
- ¼ tsp salt
- 2 eggs
- 1 tsp vanilla
- ¼ cup arrowroot starch
- 1/3 cup coconut palm sugar
- 1 tsp baking soda
- 1 tbsp butter
- ½ cup sour cream
- 1 cup grated apple
- For the topping:
- ½ cup almond flour
- 2 tbsp coconut palm sugar
- ½ tsp salt
- 1 ½ cups walnut
- 4 tbsp melted butter
- 1 tbsp cinnamon

Makes 4 servings
Set oven at 350 degrees. Coat the baking pan with butter. Make the topping. Process the walnuts in the food processor. Add the rest of the topping ingredients and blend a few more times to combine.

Wipe your food blender and add the dry cake ingredients. Blend to combine. Cut the butter into smaller chunks and add to the ingredients. Pulse until the mixture resembled pie crust.

Combine the wet cake ingredients. Add the grated apple. Add to the food processor. Pour the mixture into the baking dish and sprinkle the topping. Bake for 30 minutes until done.

Nutrient facts: 402 calories, 35 g fat, 9 g net carbs, 11 g protein

42. Paleo Egg Muffins
http://greatist.com/health/paleo-recipes-list

Ingredients and Procedures

These are just actually omelets baked in a muffin tin. You could add bits of meats, veggies, or even fruits if you like to make your egg muffins more delectable.

Nutritional Information:

Eggs can be your best friend when you are doing strenuous exercise. However, if you are practicing sedentary lifestyle (which is not recommended when you are in a Paleo program), you can still consume this 2 or 3 times a week. This is because eggs are a little high on calorie count. It is about 85 to 90 calories per egg.

However, eggs are good sources of Vitamin B12, Phosphorous, protein, selenium and riboflavin.

Another recommended easy to prepare snack is roasted sweet potato. Simply sprinkle your sweet potatoes with oil and rosemary and then roast until tender. Per cup of this would only have 180 calorie count. Plus sweet potatoes are so filling you would only need a little amount to feel satiated. Also, since these are complex carbohydrates, they tend to burn more calories during digestion.

43. Grain-free Peanut Butter Truffles

- 5 tbsp sunflower butter
- 1 tbsp raw honey
- ¾ cup almond flour
- ½ tsp salt
- 1 tbsp cacao butter
- 1 tbsp coconut oil
- 2 tsp vanilla extract
- 1 tbsp flaxseed meal
- ¼ cup chocolate chips
- Chopped almonds for garnish

Makes 14 truffles

Stir the jar of sunflower butter before using. Place the flaxseed meal, honey, almond flour, butter, vanilla and salt in a large bowl. Use your hands to stir all of the ingredients. Roll the dough into balls and place on top of parchment paper. Place in the refrigerator for half an hour. Melt chocolate chips then add the cacao butter. Dip the truffles into the chocolate and sprinkle with almonds. Refrigerate until firm.

Nutrition facts: 74 calories, 5 g fat, 3.9 g net carbs, 2.2 g protein

44. Triple Fat Fudge

Do not let the name of this dessert scare you; it will not make your three times big. The name refers to different healthy fat sources. This is a delicious treat that is perfect to serve on special occasions.

- ½ cup ghee
- ¼ cup coconut oil
- ¼ cup cocoa powder
- ¼ tsp stevia
- ¼ cup ghee or butter
- ¼ cup cocoa butter
- 1 tbsp raw honey
- 1 tsp vanilla

Makes 8 fudge

Gently melt the cocoa butter in a saucepan. Add the ghee, coconut oil and coconut spread. Stir well to combine. Add in the vanilla, stevia and honey. Whisk well to combine. Mix in the cocoa powder and whisk. Remove it from the heat and keep whisking to smooth all the lumps. Pour the mixture on a medium sized pan that has been lined with parchment paper. Place in the refrigerator for 2 hours. Once it is solid, pull the parchment paper to easily lift the fudge. Cut into small squares and serve.

Nutrient facts: 303 calories, 33 g fat, 3 g net carbs, 1 g protein

45. Blueberry Cream Pie

This is a delicious blueberry cream pie made without dairy. It looks and taste like a regular cream pie but made with wholesome ingredients.

- 3 cups almonds
- ½ cup honey
- 1 tbsp lemon zest
- ½ tsp salt
- ½ tsp cinnamon
- 2 tbsp coconut oil
- 1 tsp almond extract
- For the filling:
- 2 tsp plant based gelatin
- 2 tbsp water
- 1/3 cup honey
- 4 cups blueberries
- 1/3 cup lemon juice
- 1 can coconut milk

Makes 8 servings

Place the cinnamon and almonds in your blender and process until the desired texture is reached. Some people like smooth dough while others prefer to have some texture in it. Add the rest of the crust ingredients. Blend well to combine.

Make the filling by combining the water and gelatin together. Stir to combine. Add the lemon juice and stir. You can place the mixture on hot water if it gets to clumpy. Pour the coconut milk to a mixer. Add the honey. Whip until soft peaks form. Add the gelatin to the whipped cream. Pour it on top of the crust. Place in the refrigerator for 4 hours until it is set.

Top with blueberries and then serve.

Nutrient facts: 382 calories, 24 g fat, 40 g net carbs, 7 g protein

46. Coconut Raspberry Cheesecake

This delicious cheese cake has a beautiful dark pink color. The raspberry adds the right amount of sweetness and fruit flavor to the cake.

- 3 cups dates, soaked in warn water and pitted
- 1/3 cup coconut flour
- 1/8 tsp salt
- 1 cup coconut oil, melted
- 1/3 cup coconut, shredded
- For the filling:
- 1 ½ cups raw honey
- 1 cup coconut oil
- 6 tbsp tapioca starch
- ¼ tsp salt
- Coconut flakes for garnish
- 1 ½ cups coconut butter
- 5 cups frozen raspberries
- 1 ½ tsp vanilla extract
- Fresh raspberries for garnish

Makes 24 servings

Melt the coconut oil by placing the container on very hot water. Prepare the crust first. Preheat the oven at 325 degrees. Place the dates in a food processor. Add in the melted coconut oil. Blend until paste is formed. Scrape the sides of the processor. Mix the coconut flour, salt and shredded coconut in a bowl. Add the date paste and stir. Place in a pan and press down using a spatula. Bake for 30 minutes until it hardens a little bit.

Make the filling. Mix the cocoa butter, frozen raspberries, oil and honey in a saucepan. Place over low heat. Stir and cook until it is warm. Transfer to a blender. Mix in the salt, tapioca starch and vanilla. Blend for a minute then pour on top of the crust. Place in the refrigerator for 12 hours to cool. Remove from the pan and top with raspberries and coconut flakes.

Nutrient facts: 223 calories, 7.8 g fat, 35 g net carbs, 1 g protein

47. Brownie Magic
http://paleogrubs.com/best-paleo-brownie-recipe

Ingredients:
- 1/3 cup maple syrup
- 1 cup almond butter
- 2 tablespoon ghee
- 1 egg
- 1 teaspoon vanilla
- 1/3 cup cocoa powder
- ½ teaspoon baking soda
-

Procedure:
Whisk together the almond butter, ghee, syrup and vanilla. Add the cocoa powder and baking soda. Pour the batter into the baking pan. Bake it for 20 minutes or until the brownie is done outside but still very soft inside.

Nutritional Information:
One piece of brownie could give you as much as 180 calories. This is actually low in calories already as you can get as high as 300-500 calories per small brownie size if it is not Paleo made. Plus, Paleo brownie is also very high in Vitamin B6 and Magnesium.

48. Pineapple Coconut Bars
with Chocolate Macadamia Nut Crust

Coconut and pineapple is a delicious tropical combination that is perfect for dessert on a warm evening. It is easy to make and have a moist consistency.

- ½ cup almond flour
- ½ cup macadamia nuts
- ½ tsp vanilla extract
- 4 tbsp raw cacao powder
- 5 dates
- 1 ½ tsp coconut oil, melted
- For the filling:
- 1 cup fresh pineapple, chopped
- 1 tbsp lime juice
- 1 tbsp raw honey
- ½ tsp salt
- 2 eggs
- 1 ½ cup shredded coconut, unsweetened
- 1 tbsp vanilla extract
- ½ cup almond flour

Makes 8 servings

Make the crust. Combine the almond flour and cacao powder in a large mixing bowl. Blend the nuts in the food processor. Remove the pits and process until creamy. Add the coconut oil, vanilla and dates to the dry ingredients. Use your hands to combine the mixture. Spread it at the bottom of the pan lined with wax paper.

Make the filling. Beat 2 eggs in a bowl. Add in the pineapples, shredded coconut, lime juice, honey and vanilla. Mix with a spatula. Spread the mixture on top of the crust then sprinkle with the shredded coconut. Bake for 20 minutes at 350 degrees until done. Allow to cool before your slice.

Nutrient facts: 204 calories, 13 g fat, 11 g net carbs, 5 g protein

49. Fudgy Espresso Brownies

- 6 tbsp pastured butter
- 20 g coconut flour
- 1 cup palm sugar
- ¼ cup cocoa powder, unsweetened
- ½ tsp baking soda
- Extra butter for greasing
- 6 oz semisweet chocolate
- ¼ cup tapioca flour
- ¼ cup hot coffee
- 2 eggs
- ¼ tsp salt
- For the frosting:
- ¼ cup pastured butter, softened
- ¾ cup palm sugar
- ¼ cup pastured butter, melted

Makes 10 servings

Set the oven at 350 degrees. Grease the pan with butter and line with parchment paper. Melt the semi sweet chocolate and butter in double broiler. Add the coffee and cocoa powder. Add the sugar and cocoa powder to the food processor. Blend until the mixture is fine. Sift the coconut flour, tapioca flour, salt, sugar and baking soda. Beat the eggs then add the dry ingredients. Whisk then add the remaining wet ingredients. Pour batter into a pan. Bake for 30 minutes at 350 degrees. Allow to cool.

Make the frosting. Scoop the sugar into the food processor and blend until the mixture is fine. Heat the sugar then add the butter and coffee. Stir until it is dissolved. Place in the refrigerator for few hours. Beat in the soft butter at high speed. Spread on top of the brownies.

Nutrient facts: 175 calories, 13 g fat, 11 g net carbs, 3 g protein

Paleo Snack Recipes

One of the principles of Paleo is to cut out food not because it is forbidden but because it is not good for your body. Healthy snacks can keep you energized in between meals.

50. Tortilla Chips

These chips are good substitute for salty and crispy store-bought chips and taste delicious when paired with guacamole. It is made with wholesome ingredients so you don't have to be guilty eating them.

- 1 cup almond flour
- ½ tsp salt
- ½ garlic powder
- ¼ tsp onion powder
- 1 egg white
- ½ tsp chili powder
- ½ tsp cumin
- ¼ tsp paprika

Makes 2 servings

Set the oven at 325 degrees Mix all of the ingredients in a large bowl until you have dough. Roll the dough in between two parchment papers. Roll it out until it is as thin as you like. Cut the dough into your desired shapes. Remove the parchment paper and transfer to the baking sheet. Bake for 13 minutes until brown. Allow to cool for 10 minutes before serving with your favorite salsa.

Nutrient facts: 94 calories, 7.3 fat, 2.1 net carbs, 5 g protein

51. Sweet Potato, Goat Cheese and Kale Pizza

Pizza is one of the most popular snacks because of its delicious flavor. This is a Paleo version of the Italian pizza. It is easy to make and tastes more delicious than regular pizza.

For crust:
- 2 cups cauliflower, grated
- 1 egg, beaten
- 1 tsp oregano
- 1 cup mozzarella cheese, grated
- 1 garlic clove, minced
- For the pizza:
- 1 sweet potato, medium
- 2 tbsp goat cheese, crumbled
- ½ tsp salt
- 2 cups kale leaves, chopped
- 2 garlic cloves, chopped

Makes 8 servings

Prepare the crust. Coat the baking sheet with olive oil. Spread the cauliflower on the baking sheet and bake it for 20 minutes at 400 degrees. Combine the cheese, garlic, oregano, egg and cauliflower in a large bowl. Spread on top of parchment paper to create the crust. Bake for 25 minutes at 400 degrees.

Bake the sweet potato in the oven until it is cooked. Heat the olive oil in a pan. Add the kale and cook for 5 minutes then set aside. Remove the skin from the sweet potato and mash it to the pizza crust. Spread the garlic on top. Sprinkle cheese and kale. Bake in the oven for 10 minutes at 350 degrees. Set it aside to cool for 10 minutes before slicing.

Nutrient facts: 109 calories, 5 g fat, 6 g net carbs, 8.2 g protein

52. Peach Coconut Donut Holes

Everybody experiences sweet cravings once in a while. These Paleo snacks are made with fruits to add natural sweetness without the added chemicals and preservatives.

- 5 medjool dates, pitted
- 3 eggs
- ¼ cup coconut flour
- 1 tbsp cinnamon
- ½ tsp salt
- 1 tbsp water
- 1 tsp vanilla
- ¼ cup coconut oil, melted
- ¼ tsp baking soda
- ½ cup peaches, diced
- For the glaze:
- ¼ cup coconut butter
- 1 tsp vanilla
- 1 peach, cored and sliced
- 2 tbsp honey
- Dash of cinnamon

Makes 20 small donut holes

Preheat the donut hole maker. Mix the dates with water. Heat the mixture for 30 seconds. Remove from the heat and mash with a fork to make a paste. Add the eggs and vanilla then pour the mixture to the food blender. Add the remaining ingredients except for the peaches. Process it until all ingredients are incorporated. Add in the peaches. Add the right amount of batter to the donut hole maker and follow manufacturer's instructions.

Make the glaze by mixing the peaches, honey, vanilla, butter and cinnamon in the food processor. Let it cool then dip the donut holes into the glaze to coat.

Nutrient facts: 90 calories, 5 g fat, 8 g net carbs, 1.6 g protein

53. Power Balls

These power balls can satiate you and give you energy without using too much sugar.

- 1 medium sweet potato
- 1 tsp vanilla protein powder
- 3 egg yolks
- 2 tsp honey
- 1 cup shredded coconut, unsweetened
- 2 cups almond meal
- 2 tsp baking powder
- 4 tbsp coconut oil, melted
- 3 tbsp coconut flour

Makes 16 balls

Cook the sweet potato in a pot of boiling water. Let it cool before you peel. Mash until there are no chunks. Mix in the vanilla powder, almond meal and baking powder until everything is incorporated.

Stir all of the wet ingredients in a bowl. Add the coconut flour. The mixture should be moist and not too dry. Do not add too much coconut flour since it can absorb a lot of water. Cover the baking sheet with parchment paper. Set the oven at 350 degrees. Shape the balls into rounds and roll it in shredded coconut and coconut flakes. Chill before serving.

Nutrient facts: 141 calories, 12 g fat, 4 g net carbs, 3.5 g protein

54. Fast Crust Pizza Bites

These pizza bites are packed with pizza flavor. This is a perfect snack for children and you can serve it as often as you like without the guilt.

- ½ pack pepperoni
- 1 tbsp olive sliced
- 2 tbsp organic mozzarella
- For the sauce:
- ¼ tsp garlic powder
- ½ tsp Italian seasoning
- 3 tbsp tomato sauce
- ¼ tsp ground oregano
- ½ tsp salt

Makes 4 servings

Set the oven at 400 degrees. Line the baking sheet with wax paper. Combine all of the sauce ingredients in a bowl. Whisk to combine. Layer the pepperoni on the wax paper. Spread mozzarella cheese on top and spread 1 tsp of sauce. Top with olive slices. Bake for 3 minutes then let it cool before serving.

Nutrient facts: 134 calories, 10 g fat, 0 g net carbs, 8 g protein

55. Crispy Pretzel Snack

These pretzels are free from grains, nut and eggs so these are perfect for people with food sensitivities.

- ¼ cup arrowroot flour
- ¼ cup coconut flour
- 3 tbsp palm shortening, melted
- 1 tsp salt
- ¼ cup water chestnut flour
- 1 cup water
- 1 tsp maple syrup
- Pinch of onion powder
- Pinch of garlic powder

Makes 6 servings

Set the oven at 350 degrees. Mix all of the ingredients in a large bowl and stir until the batter is thick. It should have the same consistency as pancake batter.

Fill a pastry bag with the mixture. Cut the tip off and squeeze out pretzels by making two loops. Place in the oven and bake for 10 minutes. Let it cool before serving.

Nutrient facts: 84 calories, 7 g fat, 3.5 g net carbs, 1 g protein

56. Caveman Fries

Curb you junk food craving with this Paleo fries version. This is a great portable snack that you can enjoy while watching a movie.

- 2 lb Jicama
- ½ tsp salt
- ¾ cup raw cheddar cheese, shredded
- ½ cup mayonnaise
- ½ cup coconut oil, melted
- ½ cup onion, diced
- ½ cup mayonnaise

Makes 8 servings

Prepare your fries sauce by mixing the ketchup and mayo in a bowl. Stir it until well blended. Place in the refrigerator. Set the oven at 400 degrees and cover the baking sheet with foil. Peel the jicama and slice into fires. Rinse and pat it dry. Place in a large bowl then add the oil. Transfer to the baking sheet and spread it out. Season it with the salt. Bake it in the oven for 40 minutes until it is brown. Remove the fries from the oven and let the excess oil drip. Top the fries with the cheese and place in the oven for 5 minutes to melt. Cook the onion in coconut oil until it is golden brown. Mix the fries and onion then serve with the sauce.

Nutrient facts: 321 calories, 27 g fat, 12 g net carbs, 4 g protein

57. Healthy Fruit Leather

This is a healthy alternative to commercially bought fruit leather. This recipe also does not need dehydrator.

- 2 apples, finely diced
- 1 grapefruit, diced
- 1 tsp cinnamon
- ¼ cup water
- 10 strawberries, diced
- Stevia for sweetener
- ½ tsp salt

Makes 10 strips

Place fruits in a saucepan. Add water and boil. Simmer until the fruits are soft. Add the salt and cinnamon. Place the fruits in a food processor and blend until smooth. You can adjust the taste and add sweetener if desired. The grapefruit can taste tart so adding sweetener can balance the sour flavor.

Heat the oven to 300 degrees. Line your baking sheet with wax paper. Pour the mixture to tray and spread it evenly using a spatula. Make sure that you spread it out very thinly. Place in the oven at the lowest shelf and bake for 8 hours. Remove the tray and cut the fruit leather into strips. Let it cool before rolling it up or storing.

Nutrient facts: 27 calories, 0.1 g fat, 5 g carbs, 0.2 g protein

58. No-ritos

These are corn free Doritos made from coconut flour. It does require some effort to make but it is worth it.

- ¾ cup almond flour
- ¼ cup flax seeds
- ½ tsp salt
- ½ tsp cumin
- 1 egg
- ¼ cup coconut flour
- ¼ cup ghee
- 1 ½ tsp chili
- ½ tsp paprika powder
- ½ tsp garlic powder

Makes 4 servings

Melt the butter then transfer in a large bowl. Add the remaining ingredients and knead into a ball. Spread a baking paper on a flat surface then place the ball on top. Place another sheet on top. Flatten it with a roller then cut triangles with a knife. Set the oven at 350 degrees then bake for 10 minutes. Check it often to make sure that it doesn't burn. Let it cool for 15 minutes.

Nutrient facts: 231 calories, 20 g fat, 2.2 g net carbs, 5 g protein

59. Cajun Mini Dogs

These are great snacks for children. They are also low in carbohydrates and can be prepared in just 30 minutes.

- 12 mini sausages
- ¼ cup coconut flour
- ¼ cup grated cheese
- ½ tsp baking soda mixed with 1 tsp apple cider
- ½ tsp mustard powder, ground
- ¼ tsp salt
- 2 tsp jalapeno, minced
- 1 cup cauliflower, ground
- 2 eggs, beaten
- 1 ½ tbsp coconut oil
- 1 tbsp red pepper sauce
- 1 tsp paprika
- ¼ tsp chili powder

Makes 2 servings

Set the oven at 400 degrees. Cover the baking sheet with parchment paper. Place the cauliflower florets in the food processor and blend until it has the same texture as rice.

Place the remaining ingredients in a bowl and stir to combine. Place a spoonful on the batter and flatten with spoon. Take the mini sausage and press one dog into each section. Place another spoonful of batter on top to cover the sausage. Bake for 20-23 minutes until the top is firm. Let it cool then serve with your favorite sauce.

Nutrient facts: 137 calories, 7.5 g fat, 1.7 g net carbs, 8 g protein

Paleo Drinks

A glass or two of quality red wine is allowed in Paleo diet. You can enjoy a sip after a delicious Paleo meal. However, if you are bent on experiencing a real Paleo regimen, try the following smoothie and shake. You can't go wrong with this refreshing drink.

60. The Paleo Black Forest Shake
https://origin.ih.constantcontact.com/fs075/
1103559897241/img/78.jpg

Ingredients and Procedure:
Simply place in a blender the following ingredients: 1 cup pitted cherries, 2 tablespoon unsweetened cocoa powder, 1 cup coconut milk. Whir the ingredients until smooth. Top with dark chocolate chips, dairy free of course. And there you have it!

Nutritional Information:
A glass of the regular shake like this could cost you around 500 calories or an hour of jogging. Do not fear. This yummy Paleo black forest shake would only cost you half of that—around 200-300 calories per glass. You can enjoy this without the guilt.

Or how about this Paleo Smoothie Delight? You can mix and match any fruit that you like from banana, kiwi, and mango to strawberries. You can even invent your own smoothie by choosing your own fruits combination.

http://essentialhealth.com/2013/07/
delicious-smoothies-to-enjoy/

Procedure:
Just place the fruits of your choice (preferably 2-3 fruits only as not to produce an over tasty drink) in a high-speed blender. Then add ½ cup unsweetened almond milk and 1 teaspoon honey. Whir until smooth. Serve immediately.

Nutritional Information:
The calorie count would depend on the fruits that you add. Starchy fruits like bananas have higher calorie count. An estimated 200-300 calories is equivalent to a glass of smoothie. To lower the count, serve the smoothie on a smaller glass.

The Completeness of the Paleo Diet

A lot of positive feedbacks have been given about this most searched weight loss dietary regimen – Paleo diet. It cannot be denied that its completeness makes it more attractive and easier to its followers. The overall good results that the Paleo dieters enjoy also encourages others to find out for themselves the real score about this phenomenon.

Although the main focus of the discussion here is about the diet itself, it is for your own benefit that the following reminders be stated.

1. Intermittent fasting is included in the Paleo program. As a precautionary measure, approval from your primary health care provider is needed to ensure that you can practice fasting at least once a week.
2. The Paleo diet is to be accompanied with exercise and other activities such as sports and outdoor events. Diet alone would not give you that toned, leaner look that you are aspiring to have.
3. The Paleo diet is not the be-all, end-all of dieting. This is just a guideline to a better you. There are other things that you can include to provide you with the total wellbeing that you are targeting.
4. Do not be too hard on yourself. Once in a while, you may fail or give in to previous desires. You are a human being. Mistakes are expected to occur. However, try to get back to the program as soon as you can.
5. The Paleo diet was designed to make your life simpler and healthier. Do not complicate the simplicity of this program by trying to make it that which it is not. The Paleo diet should not make you abhor today's technology. Instead, you can benefit using the new technology to have a better health. Use technology for your advantage and not against you.

CHAPTER EIGHT:
FREQUENTLY ASKED QUESTIONS

What is the Paleo Diet?

The Paleo Diet is short for Paleolithic Diet. It is a diet based on the kinds of food eaten and how food was consumed by our ancestors who lived during the Paleolithic era. This is also called *the cavemen diet* since it is patterned from our Paleolithic ancestors who were cavemen, hunters, and foragers.

Who started the Paleo Diet?

The Paleo Diet was presumably the diet of our Paleolithic Era cavemen ancestors. However, in recent years, this diet was brought to mainstream media attention by Loren Cordain when he wrote and published the book *The Paleo Diet* in 2002. Then in 2013, Paleo became a buzzword again after it was endorsed by more people, especially celebrities and fitness gurus.

What's so special about the Paleo Diet?

The proponents of the Paleo Diet presume that during the Paleolithic era, a time lasting about 2 million years and only ended until some 10,000 years ago, our cavemen ancestors only ate and foraged for food. All these changed when planting and agriculture were developed, forcing our later ancestors to stay put to cultivate and farm their lands. However, our own genetic and nutritional makeup was still only adapted to the cavemen era settings and had not changed when agriculture came about. Due to this mal-adaptation in recently cultivated food sources like grains, legumes, dairy and other artificially-processed foods, humans developed diseases that did not exist during our cavemen ancestors' time but which continue to plague us today. By following what and how our Paleolithic era counterparts have eaten through the Paleo Diet, we will have healthier and longer lives.

So, how does the Paleo Diet work?
Firstly, Paleo works by eliminating all non-natural and processed foods in your diet. By just doing that, you'll get a host of positive results in your body and energy levels. With the Paleo diet, your meals will consist mostly of protein, a few carbs, and lots of vitamins and minerals from fruits and vegetables. Grains and artificial sugars (except from natural sources like fruits) are not allowed.

So no carbs?! None at all?
Carbohydrate-rich foods are still important. However, your body's carb requirement will be met by eating food from all-natural sources only, most notably those from fruits and vegetables.

How do I lose weight with the Paleo Diet?
As with all low carb diets, weight loss is achieved when the body's energy is used to burn fat. Typically, our body uses carbohydrates as an energy source. However, once carbohydrates are eliminated in our diets, energy is expended for burning fat instead, thus effectively reducing weight.

So Paleo means eating all-natural foods. How about milk and dairy products?
Our cavemen ancestors did not bring any cows with them as they foraged for food and look for shelter. Milk, through breastfeeding, was only for babies. Just like with grains, milk now is overly processed and filled with artificial hormones. With the Paleo Diet, doing away with all milk and dairy products is vital.

What do we eat?
We consume foods that are all naturally-occurring. This

means that the Paleo-approved foods are those that did not undergo artificial processes before they are eaten. Examples of these are meat from grass-fed animals, eggs, free-range fowl, and wild fish, natural or vegetable-sourced oils like olive oil, avocado oil, coconut oil, fruits, and vegetables.

Beef from grass-fed cattle is healthier and closely resembles that eaten by our Paleolithic ancestors back in the day. Wild fish and fowl are also encouraged since they are most likely not fed with artificial grains or feeds that are common in commercial and heavily-processed foods today.

What do we drink? Are there any Paleo milk-substitute options?
For your hydration needs, nothing beats drinking water. And yes, you can try almond milk or coconut milk instead of dairy. Others also sometimes indulge in green tea and coffee for they are rich in antioxidants.

Will eating all these not make me fat?
Not really. Yes, you will have the liberty to eat as much as you want. However, these foods are very filling that you will not feel hungry again until it's time for your next meal. The all-natural food combinations are also very nutritious.

How do I balance each meal's nutrients, serving sizes, calorie counts, and stuff like that?
The Paleo Diet nutritional plan is really simple. After all, our Paleolithic cavemen ancestors did not have to keep track of their calorie counts back then and yet they stayed lean, fit, and healthy. So just remember that for each main meal, you should include: 1) a good protein source, 2) a fruit or mixture of vegetables, and 3) some healthy fat source. That's it!

Wait. Fat? But doesn't fat make me fatter?
One of the hallmarks of the Paleo diet is its debunking of

some health and nutrition myths. One of these is that all fat is unhealthy. Everything is now labeled as low-fat or fat-free, but the human body really needs fat—healthy fats, that is.

To get optimum results with the Paleo Diet, you will need to avoid unhealthy fat sources like animal-sourced oils. Instead, use natural fat sources like fish oil, avocado oil, olive oil, etc.

Does this diet have an eating frequency or timing plan?
The good thing about the Paleo Diet is that you only eat when you're hungry, but not too hungry enough that you'd want to eat a horse. This is called Intermittent Fasting. Our ancestors who were all mostly hunters and gatherers used to do this all the time too. They couldn't always eat whenever they wanted to. They would need to hunt for game and fowl or pick wild berries or fruits before they could eat. Food was something they needed to find, not something that was readily available. They could go around looking for food for a long time before they could eat and their bodies were able to greatly adapt to this.

If I'm on the Paleo Diet, it seems I will not be eating out that much since there are no Paleo-friendly restaurants.
This should definitely not be the case. There are countless ways that you can eat out without ruining your Paleo Diet. When choosing your main dish, select a meat-based one. If possible, ask your waiter if they are able to cook the dish in olive oil or coconut oil. You can even opt to order more vegetables in lieu of your rice or pasta. Most restaurants can cater to these small and simple requests.

Can you give Paleo meat suggestions?
The basic tenet of Paleo meat selection is that the meat source should be grass or pasture-fed. Anything that has been processed like hot dogs, spam, canned corned beef, or meat loaf is a big no-no. Instead, you can try: Lamb chops, chicken (thigh, breast, and wings), bacon, eggs (chicken,

duck, etc), pork (chops, tenderloin), steak, veal (meat of young cattle), grass-fed beef, and goose.

Or you can even try your hand in getting and eating the following: Venison (meat of game animal like deer), buffalo, elk, goat, rabbit, wild boar, kangaroo, rattlesnake, ostrich, turtle, emu, reindeer, or even a bear. These are the types of meat our cavemen ancestors were definitely able to find and eat back in their days. Other Paleo meat suggestions are from seafood. You can try shrimp, lobster, clam, wild salmon, shellfish, crayfish, scallops, and crabs.

How about Paleo fish suggestions?
For fish suggestions, remember that it is always better to eat wild fish i.e. those that grow in cold bodies of water like oceans and seas. Farmed fish or those that were raised in fish ponds tend to be fed with artificial fish food and often contain higher levels of mercury. You can try eating wild salmon, tilapia, trout, shark meat, tuna, mackerel, bass, sardines, red snapper, sunfish, swordfish, cutlass, and walleye.

Now how about Paleo vegetables?
Most vegetables are Paleo. Just be mindful that some vegetables like squash, beets, and potatoes are starchy vegetables and are therefore high in carbohydrates. If you want to lose weight, it is better to look into other Paleo vegetable options instead. You can choose from a wide variety of greens like broccoli, cabbage, cauliflower, celery, Brussels sprouts, asparagus, artichoke, spinach, eggplant, green onions, zucchini, cucumber, all kinds of peppers, carrots, parsley, avocado, kale, etc.

Any Paleo fruits?
All fruits are Paleo. Just be aware of the high fructose content of fruits. Most people's favorite fruits are oranges, apples, pineapples, strawberries, lemons, watermelon, blueberry,

peaches, mango, grapes, plums, tangerines, figs, lime, cantaloupe, bananas, peaches, blackberries, dragon fruit, etc.

How about peanuts?
Nope. Peanuts are legumes and they are not Paleo. And that includes peanut butter too.

As an option, you can try other kinds of nuts instead. Try almonds, pecan, cashews, walnuts, pumpkin seeds, pine nuts, sunflower seeds, hazelnuts, and macadamia nuts.

What are other types of legumes that are not Paleo?
All legumes are not considered Paleo. So you should stay away from all types of beans like Mung, black, Fava, white, string, pinto, green, Lima, kidney, horse, Adzuki, navy, red, etc. Peas are also legumes. So stay away from black-eyed and sugar snap peas, chickpeas, and snowpeas. Other legumes and derivatives you should avoid are soy beans, soya milk, miso, lentils, tofu and mesquite.

All these things to eat, but what are the things NOT to eat while in the Paleo Diet?
Here is the general list of things that aren't Paleo and therefore you shouldn't eat: Soft drinks, dairy (all milk and milk-products like ice cream and cheese), artificial fruit juices, legumes (beans and peas), grains (oats, rye, bread, cereal, corn, pasta, etc), fatty meats, artificial sweeteners, candies, junk food, energy drinks, and alcohol.

Can you give an example of a Paleo Diet meal plan?
A good Paleo Diet meal plan will include one main protein source and one to two fruits or vegetables per meal. You can eat as many of these foods as you want until you feel full. A sample meal plan will include a serving of grilled or baked chicken or even seafood. Then you can add a garden salad and baked sweet potato if you prefer an additional natural carbohydrate source. Then, you can get an apple or orange

for dessert. Eat everything until you feel full. Please do note that if you are trying to lose weight, decrease your fruit intake since fruits can have higher amounts of calories.

Here's a full day's Paleo menu that you can follow.

Breakfast: Bacon and eggs plus one banana. (Yes, bacon from pasture-raised pork is Paleo! Woohoo!)
Lunch: Chicken salad in olive oil dressing and nuts sprinkled all over
Snack: An apple. Or a Paleo smoothie.
Dinner: Vegetable stir fry with ground beef. Add strawberries (or any berries) for dessert if you prefer.

Any suggestions for delicious Paleo snack ideas?
Snacking has never been more inventive and delicious with the Paleo Diet. You do not need to worry if you're overeating or not. You can eat anything from the leftovers of your Paleo dinner from last night, hard-boiled eggs, a fruit, nuts (except peanuts), apple slices dipped in almond butter or any butter from grass-fed cows, beef jerky, and even blueberries and coconut cream smoothie. The smoothie recipe options are endless. Feel free to be experiment on the variety of Paleo fruits and vegetables available to you and you'll come up with a new favorite Paleo snack soon.

This diet plan sounds expensive.
Getting all-natural food sources can indeed be draining on your budget. We cannot deny that organic meat and vegetables are priced higher due to the needs in growing such products away from pesticides, GMOs, and artificial toxins. A great thing now is the availability of special markets selling homegrown organic vegetables and meat from pasture fed cows or fowl and you can save on the cost when purchasing Paleo food. If you can't afford these options, choose the least processed meats or vegetables available to you. Another option is to grow your own organic garden. It

can be relatively easy, economical and sustainable enough for you and your family's natural food source needs.

The Paleo/Not Paleo food selection is still confusing.
Don't fret; there are numerous mobile apps available now that will help you identify if a food/recipe/ingredient is Paleo or not. You can download these free mobile apps for you smart phones. Getting these apps will help remove the hassle in choosing your food and instead you can focus on preparing and enjoying your meal!

I really can't give up pizza, cheese, French fries, and ice cream!
If you really, really, really can't, then don't. You can try it for a week, a month, or a few days. It will really depend on you, how you feel about your body, and you will feel after you've tried it. We all want healthier bodies and lifestyle. If the Paleo Diet can help you achieve that, then that's great!

Have heard/read/was told that this diet is bogus.
Just like any modern diet plans, the Paleo Diet also has it critiques. This ranges from the diet having no substantial scientific research backing to the diet not really working at all. It has even gotten a lot of scholars, researchers, and its proponents engage into lengthy discussions *(and name-calling)* about their own sides. But we do not want to get into that here. If the diet sounds logical to you, try it even for a few days and let's see what works.

This all still seem like a fad to me...
As an option, you can always try the 30-day or 21-day approach. Just test it out; gradually eliminate some non-Paleo foods in your diet. You do not even have to go all Paleo right away. You can have *cheat* days once a week where you eat all the French fries and ice cream that you want. Give yourself some time to adjust. Test out your energy levels each day. Do you feel any difference in the quality of your

sleep, your energy, your emotions, your hunger needs? Notice stuff like this during your trial days. Then decide.

After everything that's said, what is the main advantage of going into the Paleo Diet?

The main goal for all diet regimens is to help anyone have a healthy body. With the Paleo Diet, you will achieve this healthy body and healthy lifestyle goal without the time-consuming calorie-counting that is needed with most other diet plans. You can virtually eat any food that is considered Paleo as long you do not have specific food allergies. You do not need to constantly monitor the number of calories each serving of lamb or beef steak that you consume. You just eat whatever you like until you are full. The Paleo diet is also flexible enough for you to have days to eat a comfort food of your choice. But once you have adjusted to the Paleo diet, you will make a way to get Paleo food. Other foods just do not and will not give you the same feeling and level of energy that you have once you have been with the Paleo diet.

All these are intriguing yet logical. I want to read more or research more before I fully commit myself to this diet.

You can read Loren Corbain's book 'The Paleo Diet', Robb Wolf's 'The Paleo Solution,' or 'The Primal Blueprint' by Mark Sisson. There are countless other sources in the internet too.

CHAPTER NINE:
THE PALEO DIET: THE CONCLUSION

For some people, the Paleo diet is the answer to their prayers. Most of these people now enjoy ideal weights for their height and gender. For some, though, the Paleo diet is just one of these fads that would just cause some enthusiasm and excitement for a while and then would be gone for good afterwards.

The Paleo diet is not claiming that it is the only solution to the overweight and obesity problems of the world. However, with much commitment and adherence to the program, one could expect a full guarantee of weight loss and good health, even at 21 days only. Could you imagine how much it could do to you if you decide to continue the regimen even after the 21-day timeframe?

As with all other things, there are always two sides to the coin. You study both side of this phenomenon and decide which is the best for you.

The Good things about the Paleo diet

By removing the processed, sweetened and all artificial content in the diet, one is almost guaranteed great health. Nobody can deny the bad effects these things bring to the bodies. And yet, people still consume these, for a variety of reasons. In the Paleo regimen, the counting of calories or being strict in the serving sizes are eliminated. Eating natural and fresh foods give you the liberty to eat more and worry less.

The Paleo diet is not just about your food intake. When something guarantees you with weight loss and there are no other activities included on it, it is almost a surety that it is just a temporary fad. The "no pain, no gain" old saying stands true even today. You need exercise, good habits and a healthy lifestyle if you want a long and satisfying life on earth. There is no shortcut to a healthy life.

The Drawbacks of the Paleo diet

Although meat is allowed, grass-fed animals are the required sources of meats. That could sometimes be hard to find. Even fish should not be farm-grown. There is very little way of knowing if the meat or fish you are buying are grass fed and not farm-grown.

The tendency therefore, is just to buy the available meats on the market. There is no limitation of meat intake in this diet. However, if you have the wrong meat, you are placing your health in a more delicate state.

The Verdict

The Paleo diet has good strong points but unfortunately, there are some bad things about it too. The final say is yours, however. As mentioned in the beginning of this program, study this regimen very well before you decide to commit to it.

A study reveals that a large number of Paleo dieters follow almost 80% of the dietary program and still benefit a lot from it. However, those who benefited are those who were also active and incorporated regular exercise in their new lifestyle. You can also choose this option.

Last words for you

Start today with the intention of having a good health and a good life. The power is in you! You have what it takes to be fitter and healthier. Your journey begins today! Good luck!

CONCLUSION

Thank you again for downloading this book!

I hope this book was able to help you to understand the Paleo diet and its whole program. I also hope that you would enjoy the recipes as well as the fitter and leaner body that you are bound to have as you comply with both the dietary and activity requirements of this program.

The next step is to go and have that great health as you embark on this journey called life. The Paleo diet is one step towards the fulfillment of that dream.

Finally, if you enjoyed this book, please take the time to share your thoughts and post a review on Amazon. It'd be greatly appreciated!

Thank you and good luck!
Olivia Rose

Made in the USA
San Bernardino, CA
05 November 2016